Robert
Hope you enjoyed
The Read.
Hope I enjoy
THE STORY).
Danien
12/1/20

Forever at the Finish Line

The Quest to Honor New York City
Marathon Founder Fred Lebow
with a Statue in Central Park

Daniel S. Mitrovich

Foreword by President Bill Clinton

D1025854

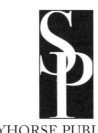

SKYHORSE PUBLISHING

Skyhorse Publishing books may be purchased in bulk at special discounts for sales promotion, corporate gifts, fund-raising, or educational purposes. Special editions can also be created to specifications. For details, contact the Special Sales Department, Skyhorse Publishing, 307 West 36th Street, 11th Floor, New York, NY 10018 or info@skyhorsepublishing.com.

Skyhorse® and Skyhorse Publishing® are registered trademarks of Skyhorse Publishing, Inc.®, a Delaware corporation.

Visit our website at www.skyhorsepublishing.com.

10 9 8 7 6 5 4 3 2 1

Library of Congress Cataloging-in-Publication Data is available on file.

Cover design by Tom Lau

Cover photos: Fred Lebow statue/Flickr/slgckgc and marathon runners/iStockphoto

Book design by Stories to Tell, www.StoriesToTellBooks.com

Print ISBN: 978-1-5107-3075-5

Ebook ISBN: 978-1-5107-3076-2

Printed in China

DEDICATION

I am grateful to God for his love and blessing in my life. When you come to understand that, your priorities change—and mine have.

For Linda; together we are an amazing team, and to our beautiful blended family.

Our children, Marissa, Heidi, Jess, Luke and Matthew, have always shown their love and encouragement towards me by running with me, asking me for advice on training programs, and listening to my ideas about the statue and now this book.

A special thanks to Anne Roberts, Scott Lange, my dearest friend Michael Crom, my brother George Mitrovich, George Hirsch, and Allan Steinfeld for their steadiness and inspiration.

To Henry Stern, the man who named me "Statue Man" and a man I call my friend.

William Jefferson Clinton for writing an introductory letter for my book and for always saying yes to support my effort in honoring Fred Lebow.

Kathrine Switzer, Kitty Kelley, and Michael Reagan for opening my eyes to what lay ahead of me in writing this book.

To Christine Robbins, for seventeen years of dedication to both Linda and me, and to Cecilia Milner who kept me on track, put up with my lack of computer skills, and demonstrated great patience in helping me write this book.

PRAISE FOR FOREVER AT THE FINISH LINE:

"After spending eighteen years in the US Senate trying to solve many problems for this fine country of ours, I thought I knew "the ropes"—but after watching my friend Dan Mitrovich try to get a statue in New York's Central Park, my efforts were "kid stuff!" After reading this wonderful book about Dan's courage and persistence, you'll know one thing for sure: there is a statue of Fred Lebow in Central Park! Here you will read what it takes to overcome huge obstacles in a quest to accomplish something of great good."

—Alan K. Simpson, United States Senator, Wyoming (retired)

"It is an inspiring story of a man whose remarkable level of determination and ingenuity enabled him to complete a most ambitious undertaking . . . If you want to be encouraged about your fellow man, this is a good book to read."

—Ronald F. Phillips, Senior Vice Chancellor & School of Law Dean Emeritus, Pepperdine University

"A perfect ending to a life well run, and a must-read for any fan of our sport—not just running, but any sport."

—Tracy Sundlun, Senior VP of Global Events for the Competitor Group and Co-Founder of the Rock'n'Roll Marathon Series

"Fred Lebow was an amazing man, the founding father of the New York City Marathon. It took another amazing man, Dan Mitrovich, to have Fred's statue created and then placed in Central Park. This is the compelling story of these two visionaries."

—George A. Hirsch, chairman of the New York Road Runners Club and former worldwide publisher of *Runner's World*

Contents

Foreword

When I was first running for President in 1992, the national press made much of my daily jogging habit. By then, I had been doing it nearly every morning for almost twenty years.

From Little Rock to Washington, and Vancouver to Seoul, I rarely missed an opportunity to lace up my sneakers. Both as Governor and as President, my runs provided a sense of routine and calm in days that were often anything but, and especially during my White House years, they were a terrific way not only to stay in shape, but to stay connected with people from all walks of life at a time when I worried about losing touch with the experiences of ordinary Americans.

Most mornings I jogged out the back gate of the White House and up the Mall to the Lincoln Memorial or the Capitol, much to the consternation of my Secret Service detail who would have preferred a more secure route. I loved these runs and enjoyed the people who joined me or who I met along the way.

As every runner knows, there are good and not so good running days. On most not so good days I chose to keep going, hoping my pounding away, regardless of the news or the weather, would provide some small measure of inspiration to joggers around the country who put one foot in front of the other for any number of different reasons. When the Secret Service finally asked me to stop running in public out of concern for my safety, I did so, but only with great regret.

Hardly anyone loved running more than Fred Lebow, or did more to turn a solitary sport into a thriving and inclusive community that welcomed enthusiasts of all backgrounds and abilities. Though few of us will ever match him in finishing sixty-nine marathons, we can all finish our run—whether a jog around the corner or a race alongside thousands of people—with a skyward nod of appreciation to Fred for sharing his incredible vision with so many of us.

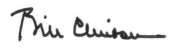

Acknowledgments

Nancy and Biff Barnes

Bobby Barrett

Nicole Burrell

John B. Emerson

Paula Rahill Fahey

Thomas Galton

Sara Katz

Bob Konlpka

Scott Lange

Cristyne Nicholas

Ken Levinson

W.A. Meston., M.V.O.

Guy Morse

Colleen Reagan

Steven Rinehart

Peter Roth

Ron Rubin

Richard Ruffner

Steve Scott

Jose E. Serrano

Alan K. Simpson

Skyhorse Publishing

Estee Stimler

StoriesToTellBooks.com

Tracy Sundlun

Ron Tabb

John Tope

Dick Traum

Special thanks to David Wimbish

Prologue
THE GREAT RACE

"In running, it doesn't matter whether you come in first, in the middle of the pack, or last. You can say, 'I have finished.' There is a lot of satisfaction in that."

—Fred Lebow

THE NUMBERS ARE STAGGERING.

100,000 applicants for 50,000 plus spots.

More than two million spectators crowding the streets of New York City.

An audience of 330 million watching on television.

No disrespect to the Super Bowl, World Series, or NBA finals, but the New York City Marathon (NYCM) is undoubtedly the world's largest and most spectacular sporting event. And unlike a Super Bowl, where fifty-three player championship rings are given out to the members of the winning team, a World Series with forty rings, or an NBA championship where there are fifteen rings, in 2016 the New York City Marathon gave out over 51,000 medals to finishers. The Marathon also raises over $340 million in revenue for the City of New York and requires the services of more than 13,000 volunteers. These include 100 linguists to assist runners from all over the world, teams of doctors, and even psychologists to aid those who run into trouble along the 26.2 mile route.

What an amazing event! And it becomes even more amazing when you consider that it grew out of a little-known run through Central Park that attracted just 127 participants in its first year, 1970.

What was it that caused this small race to blossom into the world's best-known and biggest sports event?

There's a simple answer:

FRED LEBOW

Fred was an unassuming man with a passion for running and a gift for encouraging others. He started running to increase his stamina because he wanted to improve his tennis game. But running soon surpassed tennis as the love of his life. He ran because he loved it—not for any other reason.

Fred went on to compete in sixty-nine marathons in more than thirty countries. He also served as the long-time president of the New York City Road Runners Club (NYRCC), an organization that grew from 270 members to more than 31,000 under his direction.

Tragically, Lebow died of cancer in 1994. But his vital role in making the Marathon what it is today is commemorated by a lifelike bronze statue of Fred that now greets exhausted, but exhilarated, runners at the finish line each year. The 600-pound statue is immediately recognizable to those who ran the Marathon prior to Fred's passing. They often saw him as I did, just prior to crossing the finish line. The sculpture captured the moment so well—Fred looking at his watch and shouting encouragement to runners as they gave their last few ounces of energy to reach the finish line near Tavern on the Green in Central Park.

The statue has become a New York City landmark. It is located at the 90th Street entrance to the park just off Fifth Avenue near the runner's kiosk. It's featured in dozens of tour guides to Manhattan. Every year, two days before the race, Fred's statue is moved to the finish line at 66th

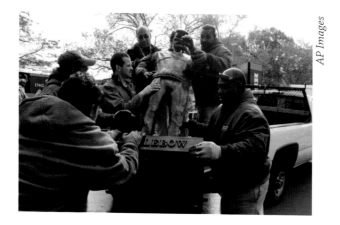

and Central Park West, and then the next day, after the conclusion of the Marathon, it is returned to its resting place near Engineer's Gate in the Park. In the days leading up to the race, it is bedecked by flowers—some from those who remember Fred and others from those who want his blessing and luck to be with them.

To look at this bronze lifelike statue, which seems so natural here, you'd never believe it took a herculean struggle to get it approved and erected in the Park—but it did. The struggle involved two United States Presidents, a governor of New York, two mayors of New York City, three United States senators, eleven members of New York's congressional delegation, dozens of celebrities, hundreds of Fred Lebow fans all over the world, and a parks commissioner named Henry Stern.

It's an incredible story and one I'm often asked to share. In fact, when people hear me talk about the statue, they almost always say the same thing: "Dan, you should write a book!"

I've heard that so often, in fact, that I finally decided to do as they suggested. The book is written, and you hold it in your hands.

Now, some people have gone so far as to claim that I "single-handedly" got the statue of Fred Lebow erected in Central Park. As I've already said, that is simply not true. The statue represents the efforts of hundreds of people. But it is true that the idea began with me and, in that sense, represents what can happen if one person has a dream and then does everything within his or her power to make that dream come true.

There are two important reasons why I decided to write this book. The first and most important reason is to honor Fred Lebow.

The second reason is to tell the story of the statue. I hope it will inspire people by showing what one person can accomplish when he or she won't give up and refuses to take no for an answer. Thomas Edison once said that "genius is one percent inspiration and ninety-nine percent perspiration." Your dream can and will come true if you give everything you've got to see it happen.

Anybody who has ever run in the New York City Marathon will tell you that the course is one of the more difficult marathon routes in the world. The last few miles may look flat to the eye, but I can tell you from experience that they are most certainly uphill. The race is grueling. But the bronze statue of Fred Lebow had a harder time getting to the finish line than any runner ever did. For over eleven years those of us who desired to honor Fred refused to take no for an answer. We fought our way through miles and miles of tangled bureaucratic red tape. And we devoted thousands of hours to keeping the dream alive.

In other words, we did exactly what it takes to accomplish almost anything worthwhile. Let me tell you how the dream began.

HOW THE ADVENTURE BEGAN

"If I can make it there, I'll make it anywhere. It's up to you, New York, New York."

—John Kander and Fred Ebb

T**HE FIRST TIME I RAN IN** the New York City Marathon, it nearly killed me.

At least I felt like I was going to die.

That was also the first time I ever laid eyes on Fred Lebow.

The year was 1990, the month was November, and the weather was unseasonably warm.

I arrived at La Guardia Airport on Thursday, November 1, at about 4:30 in the afternoon and grabbed a cab to get to my hotel, the Wyndham, at 42 West 58th Street. The Wyndham sat just beyond the side door of the famed Plaza Hotel. It was a medium-priced hotel where many of the old showbiz personalities like Donald O'Connor stayed while doing shows on Broadway. My good friends Elliot and Marjorie Martin gave me a tip on that hotel, and the hotel was a good one until it was sold several years later.

I did not jog that day, as it was my rest day. The next morning I took an early jog over to the finish line of the Marathon. I was excited just to run in Central Park and see where I would end up on Sunday. I had no idea what and how much that finish line would mean to me and how much time I would be spending there over the next eleven years.

The New York City Marathon was run on the last weekend in October through 1984. That year the weather was so hot the Marathon board decided to move the run the next year to the first Sunday in November, and there it has stayed. After returning to my hotel, I changed my clothes and got a cab to take me over to the Sheraton Hotel at 51st Street and Seventh Avenue, hoping to be one of the first to get my number and place in line. No such luck. Thousands of runners were already there, waiting in lines to get in and receive their running packets. As I made my way through the crowd, I was struck by the babble of conversation that swirled around me. Spanish in front of me. French behind me. German over there. Italian and Russian. Swahili. I knew then that this marathon was a world-class event!

Long-distance running wasn't new to me. I had been a runner since my cross-country days in high school and competed in my first marathon in my hometown of San Diego in 1981. My first marathon time was 3:54:24.

I received my official notice of acceptance into the New York City Marathon on Monday, June 25, 1990. I started training the very next day. I trained for 125 days and, for the most part, everything went smoothly. I had never trained so perfectly for a race, but this was the New York City Marathon and not just another race. When you travel all the way across the country to run 26.2 miles, you want to get the most out of it. During my training there had been a few times where my legs had cramped up about nine miles into my run. I certainly didn't want that to happen now.

On Sunday I climbed aboard one of the Marathon buses that were parked along Fifth Avenue in front of the New York Public Library, waiting to carry runners to the starting line in Staten Island. I arrived there about three hours before race time and was placed in a holding area with the longest latrine I had ever seen. There were not even separate places for women and men.

I remember that it was very cold that morning, and I made my way over to a fire truck that had its engine running so I could be warmed by the exhaust. Later that day, after the sun broke through the gray overcast, the temperature climbed to 74 degrees, making it one of the warmest days in New York City Marathon history.

As I waited for the race to begin, I noticed five other runners standing near me who were passing around a tube of some kind of ointment and rubbing it into their legs. When I started a conversation with them, I discovered that one of them had run in over fifteen New York City Marathons, another in ten, and the other three in at least five. They all looked to be in great shape. Most runners can spot other runners without any problem. These guys were tall and thin with long, strong legs built for stamina.

"What have you got there?" I asked.

The young man who had just finished greasing up his legs held the tube out in my direction.

"This is great stuff," he said. "The best."

I took it, examined it for a moment, and handed it back.

"Ever have trouble with cramping?" he asked.

I said yes and admitted that I was worried about it because I'd had some problems in my training.

"Not with this you won't," he smiled, again handing me the lotion. "Go ahead."

What could it hurt? As he nodded his approval, I squirted a big blob of the stuff into my palm and gave my legs a good massaging. Then, just to be safe, I did it again.

One thing runners learn at some point in their training for a race is that when you near the last couple of weeks prior to a big run, never, ever do anything that was not part of your overall training plan. Don't change your diet, your exercise plan, anything! Unfortunately, I had to learn this the hard way.

It was probably another half hour or so before we were escorted to the start line. Once I was at the starting line, my nerves began to kick in. I had at least 10,000 runners in front of me and another 30,000 behind me. Finally, the cannon was fired, which signaled that the race had begun—40,000 runners were on their way. Women headed to the lower level of the Verrazano-Narrows Bridge and men to the top level. There were so many of us that it would have been impossible to squeeze another human being onto that structure. Above and below, wall-to-wall—or rather, rail-to-rail—men and women of all ages and races began their run of a lifetime, the New York City Marathon.

Running through my mind was the Kander and Ebb piece, "New York, New York." We headed uphill toward the top (height of 693 feet) of that magnificent, beautiful Verrazano Bridge, 13,700 feet across. It seemed to me that I wasn't running at all. In fact, the first half-mile I was fast-walking, trying to not get knocked to the ground or trip due to the uneven road. I kept my hands on the person in front of me as I was carried upward by the momentum of the crowd. Almost without effort we reached the top of the bridge. I looked out and saw a cruise ship heading to sea. The striking view reminded me of 1968 and the first time I sailed under the Verrazano. I had been heading off to England, trying to forget the early morning hours of June 5 and the senseless murder of Robert F. Kennedy—a tragedy that shattered my life.

I continued to run down the bridge and into the borough of Brooklyn.

The next few miles came easily. I felt good, the course was flat, and the wind seemed to be at my back. I was surprised when I saw the signs for Fourth Avenue, meaning that I'd already run four miles. If only the rest of the race could go this well. As mile five and six went by, I figured maybe I could beat my 1983 San Francisco Marathon time of 3:28:37, giving me a personal best.

But as soon as that thought crossed my mind, both of my legs begin to tingle. By the time I passed the Williamsburg Bank tower, one of the tallest clock towers in the world—even taller than "Big Ben"—located near the eight-mile mark, the tingling had become a severe burning. The pain grew in intensity as I ran through Bay Ridge, Sunset Park, Bedford-Stuyvesant, and Greenpoint.

I was in agony as I drew near the Pulaski Bridge at the halfway point, 13.1 miles. The pain was nearly the worst I have ever felt. Every cell in my body seemed to be screaming for me to stop, and I had no choice but to obey.

I headed into the next first-aid tent and told the nurse my legs were on fire. She had me lie down on a little army cot and quickly began icing my legs. That ice felt great!

She shook her head sympathetically. "I don't think you're going to be able to continue. You'd better call it a day."

I actually considered it for a moment. But only for a moment. I had come almost 3,000 miles to run in this race, and I wasn't going to quit, no matter what.

After a few more minutes of rest, I dragged myself up and back out onto the street. I made it across the Pulaski Bridge into Queens and kept on putting one foot in front of the other. Somehow I managed to navigate the steep climb up to the Queensboro Bridge (also known as the 59th Street/Midtown Bridge, which Simon and Garfunkel wrote about in their song, "Feeling Groovy"). The bridge is considered one of the most difficult sections of the Marathon. We climbed about 150 feet in elevation to the center of the bridge and continued across the East River, down into Manhattan, where an amazing sea of people—at least 35,000 at that point—were waiting to cheer the runners on. The streets were absolutely full of people, cheering and shouting their encouragement, but I barely heard them. I couldn't think about anything but the pain in my legs and feet. I felt like my toes were about to fall off. I'd already been running more than three hours and still had ten miles to go.

I was in so much pain that I needed to call my daughter Marissa. I felt a desperate need to hear her voice. This was before cell phones, so I worked my way through the crowd to a pay phone and placed a collect call to Marissa, who was at home in La Mesa, California. She answered right away and I heard the operator say she had a collect call from her father and ask if she'd accept the charges. Marissa hesitated for just a moment and then said yes.

"Hi, sweetheart," I said, "this is Dad."

"Dad?" I heard the surprise in her voice. "How can it be you? I'm watching the New York City Marathon on TV right now. Aren't you running in it?"

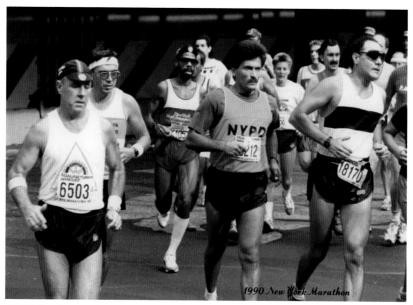

#6503 Dan Mitrovich coming off the Midtown Bridge

I told her I was but I was in so much pain that I just needed to hear her voice. I said, "I love you" and then told her I had to hang up and keep running.

I watched the street signs as I made my way up First Avenue: 60th Street, 70th, 80th, 90th. On and on I went. By the time I reached the Willis Avenue Bridge, there had been so many other runners ahead of me that the carpet they'd laid over the steel had already worn out—and the pain caused by my feet hitting that hard steel was nearly unbearable. But still I kept going.

Once across the bridge I continued to put one foot in front of the other as I headed into the Bronx, the twenty-mile mark of the Marathon. As most marathoners know, the twenty-mile mark is called "the wall." Congressman Jose Serrano told me several years later that he had asked Fred Lebow: "Why did you put the twenty-mile mark of the Marathon in the Bronx? We have enough problems here!"

Somehow I made it through the Bronx and into Manhattan via the Madison Avenue Bridge, down Fifth Avenue, where gospel singers in their choir robes brought us back to life with their up-and-moving gospel songs as we passed by.

Not too far away, a couple of blocks, perhaps, a sea of colorful autumn leaves shivered in the wind. Had I finally reached Central Park? To my great disappointment the answer was no. It was a park all right, but not Central Park. It was Marcus Garvey Park, which meant I was still almost five miles from the finish line.

By this time I was barely moving, dragging my left leg behind me. Still, pain shot through me with every step, and I was so cold I was shivering as I ran.

I had always loved running, but today I was totally, absolutely, completely miserable.

Eventually, I reached the Plaza Hotel at the corner of 59th Street and Fifth Avenue. I turned right onto Central Park South, where thousands upon thousands of spectators had gathered to cheer the runners on to the finish. Now, that was amazing! Especially considering that the fastest runners had finished the course over two hours ago. I crossed Sixth Avenue, made it to Columbus Circle, and turned into Central Park. Less than a mile to go as I moved up the last climb toward the finish line.

Then, there it was. I could see the New York City Marathon banner and the clocks showing the time. Now I knew I was about to finish.

And that's where I first saw Fred Lebow, fifty yards from the finish line, standing there, looking at his watch and shouting encouragement to runners like me. It seemed to me that he was trying to give us his own energy, willing us to finish as we came staggering towards the finish line. "Come on! You can do it!"

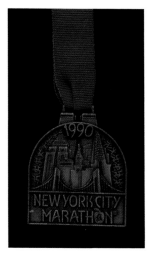

I had been waiting for so long. I had completed the Marathon in 4:39:46, far behind where I thought I'd be and wanted to be. But

1990 New York City Marathon Finishers Medal

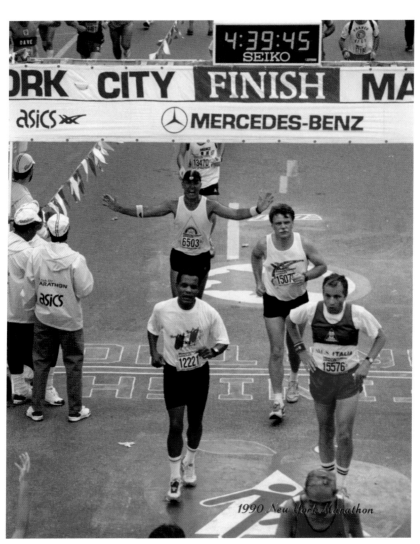

#6503 Dan Mitrovich at the finish line NYCM 1990

at least I had finished, and that made me feel so absolutely proud, I had tears of pain and happiness at the same time.

Fred genuinely seemed to care about every runner, wanted each to go home with their head held high and the ability to say, "I finished the New York City Marathon."

Olympic gold-medalist Frank Shorter put it this way:

> Fred was the only race director I knew who waved like crazy, trying to pull you in. He was so animated and excited. He couldn't sit still at the finish line. He was having so much fun because he cared about the performance. He cared about you. He wanted everyone to get out of themselves as much as possible.

I yelled Fred's name and he gave me a big thumbs up and shouted, "You did it!"

I don't know why, exactly, but that gesture and the smile on Fred's face really meant a lot to me. Just writing these words brings tears to my eyes. I knew right away that he was a very special man. If I were still alive the next day, I'd have to come back and try to meet him.

MEETING WITH THE PRESIDENT

"The pleasure, satisfaction and joy were shared by this correspondent, too! I saw that look in Fred Lebow's face— it was very touching. That was a great day for all of us."

—Alan K. Simpson
United States Senator
March 20, 1991

I F YOU COME TO MY OFFICE in Los Angeles, you'll see lots of photographs of me with famous people. Movie stars and Hall of Fame athletes, former US presidents, presidents of other countries, and political leaders from all points of the political spectrum.

I consider some of these people to be friends, and I respect and love them dearly. But I'm not in awe of them nor am I easily intimidated.

My theory is that if you approach people in the right way, they'll be happy to talk to you. In fact, the more famous they are, the more they want to talk. As they become older they want to share their stories. You just have to catch them at the right time.

That's why it was completely out of the ordinary for me to be so impressed by Fred Lebow. There was something about the guy that really spoke to me. Maybe it was due in part to the fact that he looked like such an ordinary fellow—and yet he had done such extraordinary things during his tenure as president of the New York City Marathon. The night after the race, as I lay on the bed in my hotel room, too tired and too sore to move, I decided to read some of the material I'd picked up about the history of the Marathon. The more I read, the more impressed I was.

I discovered that just a little over a year earlier, Fred Lebow had been diagnosed with terminal brain cancer. He had spent weeks in the hospital undergoing chemotherapy and radiation treatments. His doctors didn't expect him to survive more than a few months—much less return to his job as president of the New York City Marathon. But he had beaten the odds. There was no doubt that this guy was someone special.

When I woke up the next morning, the first thing I noticed was that my legs were still really sore but still connected to my body.

My second thought was, "Somebody needs to do something to honor Fred Lebow for what he's done."

I put in a call to my older brother and lifelong mentor, George, in San Diego.

"Hey, I just finished running in the New York City Marathon, and I've got to tell you, it's one of the great events of the world."

George and I have had some experience when it comes to great events. We'd gone to Super Bowls, World Series, presidential inaugurations and national political conventions for both parties. But as far as I was concerned, the New York City Marathon was the greatest event of them all. I told George about the way it brought people together from all over the world and how the whole city seemed to come together—all five boroughs: Staten Island, Brooklyn, Queens, Bronx, and Manhattan—in a spirit of friendship and cooperation on the day of the race, aptly called "Unity Day."

Suddenly, I found myself telling him all about Fred Lebow and what a great guy he was.

I said, "You know, George, I really want to take Fred Lebow to the White House and have him meet President Bush. He really deserves it." George seemed to have caught my enthusiasm. "Well, let's see what we can do about it."

As far as I was concerned, when brother George said, "Let's see what we can do about it," that meant, "Consider it done."

After the call I got dressed in my running sweats, hailed a cab, and went to the Expo headquarters at the Sheraton Hotel. I hoped to get a chance to shake Fred's hand, tell him how much running in the Marathon had meant to me—despite my unpleasant experience with that awful ointment—and ask him if he'd like to meet President Bush.

I was disappointed, but not really surprised, when the receptionist told me that I could not meet Fred and she had no idea where he was. I knew that Lebow must be exhausted after the Marathon and all the work leading up to it. I learned later that Fred most likely was at the finish line—along with Dick Traum, founder of the Achilles Track Club in 1976—waiting for the last marathoners to finish.

Many members of the Achilles Track Club, a group of runners with disabilities, might take more than twenty-four hours to finish. "If it weren't for Fred, there would be no Achilles Track Club," said Traum in the *New York Daily News* on November 3, 1994. Fred was always at the

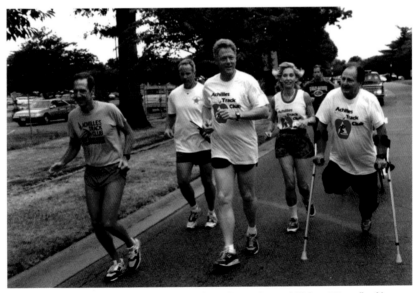

Alan Roth , Secret Service agent (left) President Clinton (center) Helene Hines (back) Dick Traum (right)

finish line to greet the runners, no matter whether they were two-hour runners or two-day runners.

I explained that I had an important message for Mr. Lebow and had hoped to deliver it personally. "Is there someone else I can talk to?"

She thought for a minute.

"Anne Roberts is here. She's very close to Mr. Lebow, and I'm sure she'll be happy to deliver your message."

I discovered that Anne Roberts served as Elite Athlete Coordinator for the New York

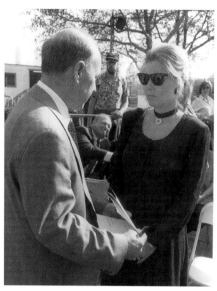

Anne Roberts

Road Runners Club. That meant she scouted and recruited world-class athletes to run in New York Road Runners Club events—such as the New York City Marathon—and she was one of Fred Lebow's closest associates, as well as one of his favorite people.

She was pleasant, gracious, and friendly, but when I told her I wanted to take Fred to meet the president, her eyes narrowed and she asked, "The president of what?"

"The United States," I explained. "I want to take him to the Oval Office to meet President Bush."

She kept smiling, but her smile seemed a little more forced than it had been just a moment ago. "That's really nice," she said. "Give us a call when you get it all arranged."

I nodded, "You'll hear from me by the end of the month."

She kept on smiling. "I'll tell Mr. Lebow."

"YOU THINK HE WAS A NUT?"

Anne delivered my message the next morning. She recalls that when she got to work that day, she found Fred waiting in her office, eating a muffin and thumbing through one of the four New York City newspapers he read every day.

He looked up as she came through the door. "How did it go?"

"I thought it went pretty well," she replied.

He nodded. "I thought so, too."

Then she said, "You know, someone kind of interesting came to see me yesterday. A man named Dan Mitrovich—from San Diego."

"What did he want?" Fred asked.

"He wanted to know if you want to meet the President of the United States—and said he would arrange a meeting for you in the Oval Office."

"Oh. You think he was a nut?"

"Probably. But he was an awfully nice man."

"Well, tell him I'd love to if you hear from him again, but you probably won't."

It was perhaps three weeks later that I called Anne, reminded her who I was, and said, "Why don't you get Fred's schedule, because the president has given us a day and time for the meeting."

She was silent for a moment and then asked, "Is this for real?"

I laughed. "It is. The president will meet us on January 31 at 3:35 in the afternoon." Then I went on. "I know what you're thinking. When I first spoke to you, you must have thought I was crazy."

"Well, I wondered," she admitted.

"But you were so nice. So polite."

"Nobody's ever rude to anybody here," she laughed. "Fred won't tolerate it."

I shared with her that Lori Rosen, scheduler for Senator Alan Simpson of Wyoming, had called with a date for the White House visit for Fred. I told Anne that Lebow should come to Washington the night before our meeting with the president. Fred, my brother George, and I would go to the leadership office in the Capitol in the morning to meet Senator Simpson, the Senate Minority Whip who had arranged the meeting for us and who happened to be, and still is, one of George Herbert Walker Bush's best friends.

JANUARY 31, 1991

January 31, 1991 came right in the middle of Desert Storm. The president had a lot on his plate, even more than a President of the United States normally does. Under such circumstances it wouldn't have surprised me if he had canceled our meeting. But he didn't. He had made a commitment to meet with us and he kept it. To me this says volumes about the President's character and integrity.

Fred Lebow was a genuine guy. There was not a single ounce of pretension coursing through his veins. This was evidenced when I saw him dressed in his dark blue, pinstriped business suit; I almost didn't recognize him. But then I looked down and saw his feet.

Running shoes.

Perfect.

I'm not really sure why Fred was wearing those shoes. However, an article written in the *Los Angeles Times* on October 18, 1991, stated: "Fred said he didn't have any dress shoes." Some people have told me that Fred always wore running shoes because hard soles hurt his feet. Others said that was just Fred. He did things his own way and was extremely confident about the way he did them.

The three of us—brother George, Fred, and I—met Senator Simpson at the Capitol, got into his vehicle—a Jeep Wrangler, as I recall—and drove the 1.7 miles to the White House. On the way I told Senator Simpson that I had brought a letter for the president from my eleven-year-old daughter, Marissa. When I'd told her that I was going to be meeting with President Bush, she had written out a short note and asked me to deliver it for her. I was a bit conflicted about the matter. I didn't want to disappoint my daughter, but at the same time, I didn't want to be presumptuous or impose on the president.

Simpson said, "Dan, let's just tell the president that you have the letter and see what he says."

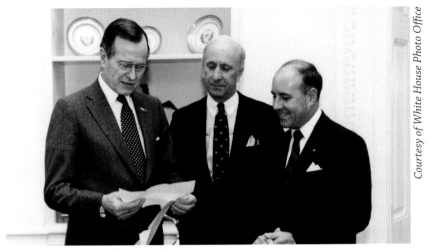

President Bush, George Mitrovich, Dan Mitrovich

From the tone of his voice, I think he already knew what would happen. (And he was right. Later, when I told the president about the letter, he immediately asked to read it. Then he sat down and wrote out a gracious reply on presidential stationery. Marissa has that letter framed and hanging on the wall in her Washington, DC office today, along with the envelope on which the president wrote, "Dear Marissa – Thanks for my letter. Your own Dad gave it to me here in the Oval Office – Good Luck Love George Bush.")

THE WHITE HOUSE

Because of the Gulf War, the city was on high alert, and this was especially true at the White House.

After being questioned and having the senator's car searched, our driver entered the White House grounds from Pennsylvania Avenue and drove us up to the West Wing. We were escorted into the lobby where we picked up our appointment badges, made a left turn, and walked down a hallway past the Roosevelt Room toward the Oval Office. The Roosevelt Room is named for both Roosevelts—Theodore, who had the West Wing built in 1902 and had his office here, and Franklin, who

THE WHITE HOUSE

Marissa

courtesy
Your own Dad

 THE PRESIDENT

1-31-91

Dear Marissa —
Thanks for my letter.
Your Dad gave it to me
here in the Oval Office —
Good Luck Love
G. Bush

President Bush's note to Marissa and envelope

27

remodeled and expanded the West Wing during his first year in office. As I thought about all the history-making meetings that had taken place here, patriotic pride welled up in my chest. I also felt pleased that a man like Fred Lebow, a great American born in Romania, was about to be honored here.

We reached the end of the hallway and turned right toward the office of the president's personal secretary and the Oval Office behind it. Senator Simpson led us into the secretary's office. Someone who looked awfully familiar was sitting there waiting to meet with the president. He stood up and greeted Senator Simpson as we walked through the door.

"Bob, good to see you," Senator Simpson said, extending his hand to Bob Dole.

Senator Dole smiled when he saw Fred's running shoes and remarked, good-naturedly, that he'd never before seen a pair of shoes like those in the White House.

In those days it may have been true that you didn't see many running shoes in the White House, but all that changed when Bill Clinton took up residence there and made running—and running shoes—fashionable. His successor, George W. Bush, also an excellent runner, kept running shoes in style when he took up residence, as well.

We chatted for a few minutes then were told that the president was ready for us, and we were escorted into the Oval Office—ahead of Senator Dole.

President Bush was as gracious and kind as he could be, and there's only one thing I regret. As the White House photographer was about to take a picture of him and Fred, the President asked me, "Dan, do you want to step into the picture?"

"Mr. President," I said, "Thank you very much, but this is Fred's moment." I've regretted ever since that I said no. Although I have a photo of me alone with President Bush, and another of George and me with the President, I don't have a picture of me with Fred and the president. This caused problems down the road, as having the photo with Fred would have been worth more than a thousand words.

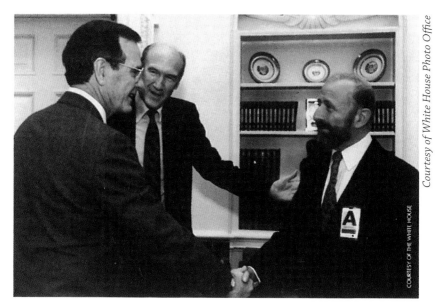

President Bush and Fred Lebow

We spent about fifteen minutes in the Oval Office, chatting with the president, who made us all feel that nothing was as important to him as we were at that moment. I was amazed by the president's patience and good nature, especially considering everything else he had on his plate. We could have been in and out of his office in five minutes, but instead, we had a nice, leisurely visit, which included a funny story Senator Simpson asked the president to tell us about Queen Elizabeth whom he took as his guest to a Baltimore Orioles game. It was extraordinary to say the least.

The story the president told us was "He has Four Balls." One of the Oriole batters got a base on balls, dropped his bat, and was walking to first base. Her majesty asked, "Mr. President, why is that man walking?" "Because he has four balls." Her Majesty responded with, "That must be frightfully uncomfortable."

The president also presented each of us with presidential cufflinks and a tie clasp.

After our meeting, on our way back to Senator Simpson's office, I told Fred I wanted to put together a luncheon for him during Marathon week

ALAN K. SIMPSON
WYOMING

United States Senate
Assistant Republican Leader
WASHINGTON, D.C. 20510

March 20, 1991

Daniel Mitrovich
9165 Grossmont Boulevard
La Mesa, California 91941

Dear Dan:

That was a beautiful letter of February 8, and
I loved having it.

The pleasure, satisfaction and joy were shared
by this correspondent, too! I saw that look in
Fred LeBow's face -- it was very touching. That
was a great day for all of us.

I will share your letter with the President,
together with the article from The Californian. He
will love it! He does not often get to see the
follow-up to his marvelous generosity and
kindness. He is a special man -- but you know that
so well.

It was good to hear from you, Dan. Keep in
touch.

Ann joins in sending our love to you and to
all of your family.

Most sincerely,

Alan K. Simpson
United States Senator

AKS/emm

that year and bring in leaders from the corporate world to honor him. I said, "If you agree, I will need two things from you. First, you need to be there, and second, I will want the banner of the New York City Marathon for the luncheon room."

He smiled and said, "Dan, you got me in to see the President of the United States. I think you can do anything."

3

NEVER GIVE UP

"Dan Mitrovich was a West Coast man, wanting to do something in New York City—with all the red tape that we have in this town—to get something in Central Park, which nobody can touch. And some people thought he was out of his mind. But he was standing tall inside. He was very, very bold. And he kept at it... And so the message of the day is, The Time Has Come. Do it."

—Dr. Arthur Caliandro, Senior Minister,
Marble Collegiate Church, New York, New York
Sunday Sermon, November 4, 2001

A S I SAT IN A PEW in Marble Collegiate Church with my wife, Linda, my daughter Marissa, and her friend Ben Beers, listening to the eloquent voice of long-time senior minister, Dr. Arthur Caliandro, I was shocked and, at the same time pleased, to hear my name mentioned. And I was even more shocked that Dr. Caliandro not only believed I had done something that would serve to turn unfulfilled dreams into reality, but the previous day's ceremony in Central Park to dedicate the Fred Lebow statue had moved him to go home that night and write a sermon inspired by my actions.

On that late autumn day in 2001, ten years after I had the idea for a statue to honor Fred, Dr. Caliandro said, and I quote:

"The day before the marathon, the New York City Marathon, which is happening as I speak, I took a small part in a very big, dramatic moment. I was present at the finish line for the dedication of the statue of Fred Lebow. Fred Lebow, you know, is the man who started the Marathon and got it going. In 1970, the first year of the New York City Marathon, it had 127 runners. Presently, there are more than 51,000 runners from different countries, and one of the speakers yesterday spoke about running needing no language. Running was running, and you could run no matter what your language was. And Fred Lebow not only started something in New York and in America, the largest and the greatest marathon in the whole world, but he ignited something for the entire world, where now a marathon is a part of every nation's culture. It's become a very big thing. He had a dream. He believed. He was bold. Brazen. And he made it happen. Dan Mitrovich was bold, he was brazen, and he made it happen!"

I believe that anyone who perseveres in pursuit of a dream can achieve it. I've never been one to take no for an answer, and if you have that attitude, there are very few limits to what you can do. Certainly, no one who has accomplished great things in life ever started out thinking, "I can't do this." They believed in themselves and in their dreams.

Experience has taught me that life is all about going around roadblocks and leaping over hurdles. If it seems the rules are against you—well, rules are made to be broken. Write new rules as you go along. If you think you can ... you can.

Over the last forty-six years, more than 1.3 million people have found out what they can do by pushing their bodies and minds to the limits of their endurance. They have done it on the streets of New York City the first Sunday in November.

THE MARATHON'S ANCIENT ROOTS

Marathon runners are taking part in an event that dates back nearly five hundred years before the birth of Jesus—to 490 B.C. The race draws its name from the Battle of Marathon, which occurred that year.

According to legend, a messenger named Pheidippides ran about twenty-five miles, from Marathon to Athens, to announce the Greek victory. He gave his one-word message, "Victory!" and then collapsed and died on the spot.

When the first modern Olympics were held in Greece in 1896, Pheidippides was honored with a race of 24.85 miles, from the town of Marathon to Olympic stadium in Athens. Only nine runners completed the marathon, and eight of them were Greeks. Sixteen others failed to finish, including the only American competitor, Arthur Blake, who dropped out after about fifteen miles. Blake had won the 1500 meters just a few days earlier. The marathon gold went to Spiridon Louis, a Greek postal worker, who crossed the finish line more than seven minutes ahead of the silver medalist.

The very next year the first American marathon took place in Boston on April 19, the third Monday in April, the anniversary of Paul Revere's famous midnight ride.

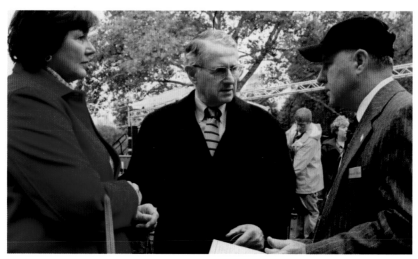

Linda Mitrovich, Dr. Arthur Caliandro, Dan Mitrovich

The original distance of the marathon was 24.85 miles. However, in London, during the 1908 Olympics, the marathon began in front of Windsor Castle, and from Windsor Castle it was exactly 26.2 miles to the royal family's viewing box at White City Stadium. For the next sixteen years, a debate raged regarding the marathon's proper length. Then, during the 1924 Olympics in Paris, the official distance was set at 26.2 miles. I will tell you, as a runner I would much rather stop at 24.85 miles than 26.2!

Since it was the royal family who brought us runners the extra mileage, I checked to see if any member of the royal family had ever run a full marathon and found none, with the exception of a distant cousin by the name of Sir Ranulph Fiennes. Sir Ranulph is an English adventurer and is known as one of world's greatest living explorers, as well as a holder of several endurance records.

In 2003 he completed seven marathons on six continents in seven days. Saving the best for last, he finished his seventh on November 1, 2003, in the New York City Marathon with a time of 5:25:46. The other six marathons were in Patagonia, Falkland Islands, Sydney, Singapore, London, and Cairo.

I found only two things Sir Ranulph and I have in common. We both love running and we were both born in 1944. He was never knighted by the Queen but is called Sir because he is a Baronet. I think the Queen should actually knight this gentleman.

FALLING IN LOVE WITH RUNNING

It was during my sophomore year in high school that I discovered the joy of running—and long-distance running, in particular. My first year at El Cajon Valley High I played freshman football. I was one of the smaller kids on the team, but I was pretty fast. At the end of practice, the coach made us run two laps around the track, and most of the time I led the group.

One afternoon during my freshman year, as I was finishing my laps, a man came up to me as I walked off the field. I didn't know who he was, although I had seen him once or twice around the P.E. facility; the cap he

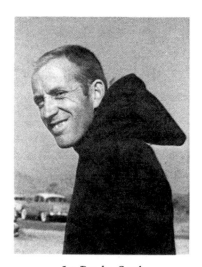

Joe Brooks, Coach
Humm—We won again!

wore and the whistle around his neck identified him as one of the coaches.

"You're pretty fast," he said.

"Thank you," I smiled.

"But why are you killing yourself out there with those big guys? Why don't you come run cross country for me? I'm Coach Brooks, and I'd love to have you run with one of my runners and see how well you do."

Coach Brooks had my attention. First of all, it made me feel good to know that he wanted me. And secondly, football was not doing it for me—and I was not that great at it. I could pass well, but I was so much shorter than my competition. I told him I'd think about it.

Not wanting to do this alone, I got my friend Dan Cary to join me. That was as simple a decision for Dan Cary as it was for me, as his 104-pound body took as much damage as mine did in football. Even with that it wasn't easy to give up football. My brother Bill was the quarterback for the varsity team, and I know he wanted me to try to be as good as he was. And I was expected to follow in his footsteps—especially by my father. The problem was that I was not nearly as big as Bill. When I finally decided to quit football and run cross country, my dad was furious. "Any jackass can run," he said.

Not exactly the encouragement I was looking for.

But Joe Brooks was a great coach who believed in us and taught us how to do our best.

Morley Field in San Diego was one of my favorite cross country runs in competition. One of the reasons I liked it so much was that it was a very steep, hilly course. Starting at the top of the hill, we would run down into the canyon and along Pershing Drive. Then we would start back up the hill. Near the end there was a very steep part that could take the strongest competitor's breath away. Once you reached the top, you had another quarter-mile or so to reach the finish line. Coach Brooks told me, "When you get to the top, dig down deep and give it everything you've got for the next 110 yards. Remember, everyone in the race is experiencing the same thing you are. Once you reach the 110-yard mark, you'll start to regain your breathing—and by then you'll have overtaken many of the other runners."

More than anyone else, he's the one who taught me that a little bit of extra effort will get you over the top and give you a better shot at victory. I spent the rest of that season, and one more, running for coach Brooks, who, I believe, was one of the great high school coaches in the history of cross country. He taught me to never give up.

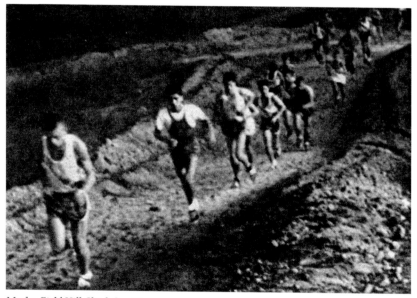

Morley Field Hill Climb San Diego

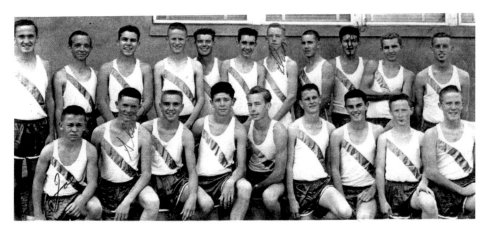

Junior Varsity: front row, left to right: Joe Heisler, Jim Andrews, John Nimesgern, Steve Johnston, Bob Applegate, Gary Hogsed, Bob Reed, Dan Connors, Tim Goebel. Back row: J.ohn Pescoe, Leon Wise, Duncan Penman, Joe Cotham, Bob Boyce, Doug Miles, Dan Cary, Dan Mitrovich, Mike Morris, Dave DeNure, George McKeon.

El Cajon Valley High JV Team Photo

THE GATHERING 1817-1968

"The man who can drive himself further once the effort gets painful is the man who will win."

—Sir Roger Gilbert Bannister

SEPTEMBER 7, THE FIRST SATURDAY OF September 1968, found me in the highlands of Scotland where the Gathering of the Braemar Royal Highland Society was taking place at The Princess Royal and Duke of Fife Memorial Park. I was intrigued by the long and colorful history of these games, which date back several centuries.

I was also enthralled by a description of the way the games begin—with a lone piper making his way down from the nearby hills, picking up followers as he passes through tiny hamlets on his way to the town of Braemar. The whole thing sounded just about perfect to me.

As I read the program of events, I discovered #23 in the program: Race, 1 mile, Handicap, Men, Open. The race would be run on the grass field in front of the Royal Box, where Her Majesty, Queen Elizabeth II, and her husband, Prince Philip, Duke of Edinburgh, would be seated. The race was open to all comers, provided you could prove you had some running ability.

I immediately tracked down an official and gained entry to the event. I was excited about running in front of Queen Elizabeth II and Prince

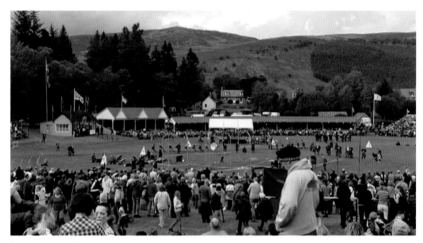

The Braemar Gathering

Philip. However, a runner standing next to me asked if I knew who the runner standing immediately to my right was. I replied I had no idea and then he said it was none other than Roger Bannister.Now, to this day, I never did confirm that the man to my right was Roger Bannister. In fact, when I asked Steve Scott about the possibility, he said it would have been highly unlikely. I have sent messages to one of Bannister's sons, Thurstan Bannister, but as of this writing have had no response.

Bannister was and is a running legend and the first man to run a mile in under four minutes, clocking 3:59:04 in May of 1954. If it *was* Roger Bannister, he would have been thirty-nine years old and most likely would not have been setting any records. (I say this even though my friend Steve Scott, former American record holder in the mile, would have broken the four-minute mile at age forty had he not been derailed by a battle with testicular cancer.) Steve Scott ran 136 sub-four-minute miles, more than any other runner in history. Still, it was a thrill for me to be running this race with the possibility that Roger Bannister was there as well. He would be knighted in 1975 for his services in medicine.

Prior to sending my book off to my editor, I communicated with the Secretary of the Braemar Royal Highland Charity, W.A. Meston, M.V.O., about that race and I asked the question: Was there any record of Roger Bannister running in it? To my disappointment, there was no official record of Sir Roger in that event.

The Braemar Gathering began in the eleventh century when clans from throughout Scotland came together for several days in early autumn to hunt deer.

Today the Braemar Gathering remains one of the world's foremost athletic spectacles, with legions of pipers, hundreds of men in colorful kilts, representing clans from throughout Scotland, members from the British Royal Family, and thousands of spectators coming together to cheer on athletes taking part in sixty-six events. These events include Highland dancing, putting the stone, and a tug of war between various branches of the British military.

Just the thrill of running in front of the Royal Box where Queen Elizabeth II and Prince Philip were seated was enough of a victory for me.

REDISCOVERING RUNNING

Over the next few years, I managed to let running slip away from me. Strange, because I had always enjoyed it so much. Still, life was so busy working at ABC Studios in Hollywood and on the road for two years touring seventy-two cities with the Disney on Parade show. Performing in ten shows a week, and then traveling to the next city, left little time for running.

Some of us runners can find many excuses not to lace up our running shoes, and I am no exception. I worked such long days that it was hard to find the time to do things that I really wanted to do—like run.

It wasn't until 1974, in Washington, DC, that I rediscovered running. When I did I wondered how I ever could have let it fall by the wayside. What a thrill it is when those endorphins start flooding through your brain—and you feel your body getting trimmer, fitter, and healthier.

There are some great places to run in our nation's capital, and I made good use of them. Washington truly is one of the most beautiful cities in the world, with all of its monuments and its ornate architecture.

Plus, everywhere you go in the city, you see something that has played an integral part in history.

One of my favorite running routes in the District took me up 15th Street to Constitution Avenue. From there I'd head up the hill to the Washington Monument. After circling the monument I'd head down across the Mall to the Jefferson Memorial, up the steps and then back down around the Tidal Basin, and along the polo fields to the Lincoln Memorial. How inspiring it was to run around the Washington Monument and up and down the steps of the Jefferson and Lincoln memorials. Beyond the Lincoln Memorial I'd pick up speed again as I'd turn left and head toward Georgetown University. I'd run up and touch the door of the main building, then turn and head back down to M Street. From there my route took me along Pennsylvania Avenue and past the White House, finishing up near 15th Street.

One of my other running routes took me up the steps of the Capitol, over to the Supreme Court building, across to the Library of Congress, and back down Independence Avenue. I also liked to run along the George Washington Parkway and through the streets in Georgetown, although you have to be careful on the cobblestones, as they can be murder on your feet and cause you to stumble.

Running from the rowing club in Alexandria along the Potomac to Indigo Landing is also one of my favorites, and I still run that run whenever I am in DC, even today.

For the next few years, I just ran for my own personal pleasure. I didn't run in any events. I didn't even keep a running diary until 1979.

RUNNING DIARIES

I have kept a running diary every year since 1979. When writing this book I referred to them constantly, as my running diaries are so accurate and tell the date, time, place, and other important notes about what happened to me on that day.

If you take nothing else from this book, make certain you start keeping a running diary. It may well be one of the more important things you do as a runner.

Running diaries are important to us runners, as they are the only way you can really compare accurate data on your history from year to year as a runner. You can track all your miles from year to year. A running diary allows you to record not only your running times of various races, but also your running times in your everyday running. You can track your weight, weather, how you feel, or if you had any illnesses.

Also, if you were traveling or you had an extreme early start in work which kept you from getting your run in, you will be able to understand why you did not run on that certain day.

Other things I often record are things like when I went to bed: not getting proper sleep can often cause you a slower time the next day. I also record any stress that may have been going on in my life with family, co-workers, or just business in general.

Normally, your time on your daily running routine—repeating the same run as you did the day before—will not vary much. As an example, if you run five miles, your time will most likely be within one minute of your previous time. It is really exciting when you take more than a minute off your previous run. You can feel really good about yourself, and it will help you the next day as you go out with a positive attitude.

I prefer running diaries that allow more space to record more of what went on in any given day. Most of the running diaries you buy have an accurate count of fifty-two weeks, so they do not give you much room to screw up on your recording. I am not certain why the publishers limit the pages; I think they need to add more pages.

Most of us runners know we most likely will not be breaking any running records, but we feel really good when we beat some of our earlier times. Remember, your running is for you; don't worry about the other runners.

By 1979 I had come back home to San Diego, where I ran regularly with my brother Bill and my friend from age five, Rick Bostrom.

Bill and I had many great times running together. I'll never forget the La Jolla Half-Marathon, which started at the Del Mar Race Track and finished at the beautiful La Jolla Cove. We were about two miles from the finish line when I started wondering where Bill was. I looked around for the running hat he always wore but didn't see it anywhere. Bill was an excellent runner, and I figured he was so far in front of me that I'd never catch him. Actually, he was about fifty yards ahead and had taken off his hat so I wouldn't see him. He didn't want to give me any incentive to pick up my pace—and possibly catch him. We were closing in on the finish line when I finally saw him. I summoned up every bit of energy, and ran as fast as I could, but fell a few yards short of catching him.

Although Bill had many faster times than I did, I still have the overall best times for the 13.1-mile half-marathon and the 26.2-mile full marathon.

It was Bill and our good friend George Cretton who first got me interested in running a marathon. Although Coach Brooks had told me about the Boston Marathon many years before, it took Bill and George to get me to start thinking I could actually keep going for 26.2 miles. They had successfully completed the 1980 San Diego Marathon, and I had been there to cheer them on.

At that time marathon running was still something fairly new; only about 143,000 runners were running marathons in America in 1980, compared to about 550,000 in 2016. The running boom had yet to take off, and I wasn't really sure I could do it. But, as it turned out, when I did run my first marathon in San Diego, I enjoyed the physical thrill that came from pushing myself to the limit.

Although I was born in San Diego and had spent much of my life in the area, running a marathon in your hometown will open up a totally different way of looking at your city. In 1981 the San Diego Marathon began on Coronado Island, came across the two-mile-long San Diego-Coronado Bridge that spans San Diego Bay, passed through Barrio Logan along the waterfront on Harbor Boulevard—passing the tall ship, *Star of India*—and continued out to Point Loma. From there the route would take you along Nimitz Boulevard out to Mission Bay, turn on Friars Road across Highway

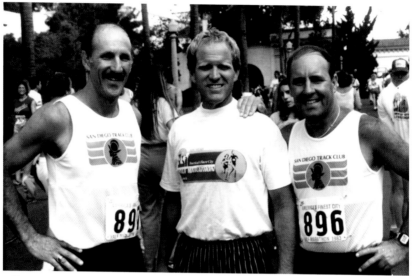

Bill Mitrovich, Rick Bostrom, Dan Mitrovich

163, and end at Jack Murphy (now known as Qualcomm) Stadium.

By the time I reached the stadium during that first marathon, the temperature had reached a sizzling 103 degrees—very unusual for San Diego. I saw lots of army cots with runners laid out on them, as the temperature took its toll on all of us that day. Despite the heat, I finished in 3:54:24, which pleased me, since my goal had been to finish in under four hours. Of course, for us runners, having someone waiting for you at the finish is one of the best parts. My wife and two-year-old daughter were there to greet me.

When I entered the San Diego Marathon, I figured it would be a one-time deal. It would be great to be able to say I'd done it, and that would be the end of it. I'd never feel the need to run in another marathon.

Wrong!

I've talked to many runners who've told me the same thing: When you come across that finish line, your body is yelling at you, "You'd better not try this again." But as soon as you regain your strength, you start thinking that you could actually do this thing again. That's exactly the way it was with me, although I didn't participate in another marathon

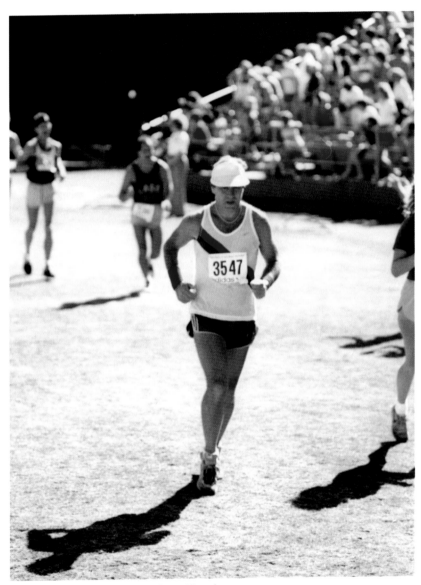

#3547 Dan Mitrovich, 1981 San Diego Marathon

until two years later in San Francisco.

The San Francisco Marathon is one of the more challenging events I've done. First, a lot of the course is uphill. In 1983 the race began in Golden Gate Park, and, eventually, you would run through the financial district and through Chinatown. Second, it can be cold in San Francisco, even in the middle of summer.

That year the marathon was held on July 24. I was in my final two miles as I ran along the wharf and made my final turn on Market Street, heading up to City Hall and the finish line. When I made that turn, my legs were just about frozen, and by the time I crossed the finish line, my body was close to hypothermia.

Nevertheless, I finished in just over 3:28:37, my personal best.

After San Francisco I kept on running, taking part in 10Ks, half-marathons, full marathons, and many other events of various lengths.

Over the years since I started keeping records, I've run 10 marathons, 17 half-marathons, and 27 10K runs. My most miles logged was in 1983, as my running journal for that year shows 1,402 miles run. I am really proud of those miles since that is an average of almost four miles a day, and for someone like me, who lives a very complicated professional life, that is one hell of a lot of miles.

An interesting note is that Fred Lebow's most miles run in one year was 2,500 miles!

A STATUE FOR FRED

"At Dale Carnegie we like to recognize individuals who show great vision. As a company that was founded here in New York City back in 1912 at 112th Street, we feel that Fred Lebow has recognized the true vision of New York. It was our honor to be involved from the very beginning, and we recognize that vision here today,"

—Michael A. Crom, Vice President of Dale Carnegie & Associates

I KEPT RUNNING THROUGHOUT THE REST OF the '80s, picking up the pace in 1990 when I decided to enter the New York City Marathon. Of course that's when I met Fred Lebow, if only momentarily. And as I stated earlier, a few months after that, on January 31, 1991, Fred, my brother George, Senator Simpson, and I met with President George H. W. Bush in the Oval Office, and that is when I told Fred about the luncheon idea I wanted to hold for him. I told him it would be that same year, just before the New York City Marathon.

As soon as I got home to San Diego, I called my friend Michael Crom, Executive Vice President of Dale Carnegie & Associates. Michael is Dale Carnegie's grandson, and his father, Ollie, served as the organization's President and CEO. I felt that Fred Lebow exemplified all the core values Dale Carnegie had always stood for—such as caring about others and refusing to let worry keep you from living life to the fullest. For that reason I believed the Carnegie organization might want to get involved in hosting an event in Fred's honor. Michael agreed with my assessment and asked me to call his father, which I did immediately. He, too, was impressed with Fred's story and asked me to get back to him with more specific information as soon as I had it.

A few weeks later I got a call from Anne Roberts.

"Dan," she said, "I wanted to let you know that Fred and I are coming to Los Angeles."

"You are? That's great! When?"

"We're coming out in March for the LA Marathon," she said. She went on to explain that they would be attending a VIP event at the Bel-Air Country Club, and Fred wanted her to call me and invite me up.

I was happy to hear the news and told her I'd make plans to drive up so I could spend some time visiting with them.

"I know Fred will be pleased," she said and then added softly, "I wanted to let you know that Fred's not feeling too well." She said she didn't know the prognosis but that Fred had been experiencing some dizziness and fatigue.

It was as if I'd just received bad news about a member of my family. I also felt a renewed urgency about my plans to honor Fred with the luncheon in New York City. Fred had beat cancer before, and I, too, believed he could do it again. But I was also concerned, and I wanted to honor him while he was well enough to enjoy the moment.

WHY NOT A STATUE?

A few weeks later, on March 1, 1991, while I was driving from San Diego to Los Angeles to see Fred and Anne, a strange thought came into my head: Fred should be honored with a statue. The idea just occurred to me out of the blue. I don't know where it came from, really, unless it was tied to all those hours I had spent running through the streets of our nation's capital and seeing all the beautiful monuments and statues there.

As soon as I walked through the door of the Bel-Air Country Club, Anne came over to say hello.

"Glad you could make it, Dan. I know Fred will be happy to see you." She looked around the crowded dining room, trying to locate him. "Now, where did he go?"

"We'll find him," I said. "I wanted to talk to you first, anyway."

"There he is!" She had spotted Fred in a corner of the room, engaged in a spirited conversation with Dr. Bill Burke, president and co-founder of the LA Marathon.

"You said he's not doing too well?" I asked.

She nodded. "Some days are better than others."

It looked like one of those good days to me, and I told her so.

"He's in his element," she replied. "Talking about running makes him forget he's sick."

"Thank goodness for that," I said. "Listen, there's another reason I wanted a few moments to talk to you."

"Which is...?"

"I've got a great idea. I want to create a statue of Fred."

"A statue?"

"That's right," I nodded. "A life-sized statue, and we'll put it in Central Park."

For a moment she looked at me as if she thought I were crazy. Then, suddenly, her entire face seemed to light up.

"I love it," she laughed. "Of course, Fred will hate the idea, but the rest of us will love it." She paused a moment and then added, "Do you really think you can do something like that?"

"I know I can," I replied.

"How?"

"I don't know," I admitted. "I'll have to find out when I get home. But let's keep it a secret for now."

"Of course."

Fred was just terrific to me, but I did notice that, although he tried to act as if everything were fine, at times he seemed a bit unsteady and slightly confused. I had a wonderful time visiting with him, and he introduced me to Dr. Bill Burke. I had previously met Dr. Burke's wife, the former Congresswoman Yvonne Brathwaite Burke, many years previous through my brother George. But this was the first time to meet Dr. Burke. He invited me to stay over and attend the L.A. Marathon the next day as his guest.

The first running of the LA Marathon was in 1986, just two years after the Los Angeles Olympics.

The next day I attended the marathon and watched as Mark Plaatjes won the Men's Open Division in 2:10:29 and Cathy O'Brien won the Women's Open Division in 2:29:38. The Men's Wheelchair Division was won by Jim Knaub in 1:40:43 and the Women's by four-time winner Connie Hansen in a time of 1:57:11.

By the time I hit the road back to San Diego on the following day, Sunday, I was deeply worried about Fred, and I also now had to think about what I told Anne the night before: that I could put a statue of Fred in Central Park.

FINDING THE SCULPTOR

"If you know Dan Mitrovich, you know that he can be very tenacious. If something is really important to him, he gets it done."

—*J. Oliver Crom, President and CEO of Dale Carnegie & Associates*

I KNEW I HAD GIVEN MYSELF A tough assignment—to commission a life-size sculpture of Fred Lebow and have it placed in Central Park to honor him—but I didn't know how tough. I had no idea of all the obstacles that had to be overcome to actually accomplish it.

Before Fred's statue could become a reality, I'd have to dig through miles-deep layers of bureaucracy, wear out dozens of scissors cutting red tape, raise the money for the statue, handle the logistics, and win support from thousands of Fred Lebow fans around the world. But working through all of that came later. Right then I knew I had a great idea and I believed I could get it done. I wasn't exactly sure where or how to begin, but I'd never let that stop me before.

I finally decided that the first thing I had to do was find a good sculptor—after all, the statue would someday stand in the most famous park in the world! The sculptor had to be someone who could portray the strength and dignity of Fred Lebow. Second, and at the time the most important, I had to find out how much it would cost to get a statue made.

This was during the days before the Internet, so I had to dial away, calling everyone I knew who might possibly know something about sculpting. Nobody had much advice to offer.

I even looked in the Yellow Pages under sculptors and statues, but I didn't get any promising leads from the few numbers listed there.

FINDING THE SCULPTOR

After that I started calling museums and art galleries throughout the San Diego and Los Angeles areas. Now I was getting somewhere.

I even got some estimates—and most of them were well over $100,000.

Was I shocked? You bet! $100,000-plus for a bronze statue? I had no idea it was going to cost that much. Even so, I never considered dropping the idea. Fred deserved it, and I would do whatever it took to get it done.

That's when I remembered my friend Tom Hazard. His grandfather, Roscoe E. "Pappy" Hazard, created a contracting company in San Diego in 1926. From cattle to construction, he did it all. His contributions to the city are memorialized in numerous ways, including a bridge dedicated to Pappy in 1970. And in 1990 the Hazard family created Hazard Center. Right in the middle of it stands a statue of Pappy, and just across from Pappy stands the statue of Tom's father, Bruce R. Hazard.

I called Tommy and asked, "Who built that statue of your grandfather at Hazard Center?"

Tommy said he knew the sculptor was a professor of art at San Diego State, but he couldn't remember the man's name. He did remember that the statue was commissioned by the developer of the property.

Prior to calling the developer to get the sculptor's name, I drove out to Hazard Center to get a good a look at that statue.

When I got there I was pleasantly surprised and excited. The statue was even better than I remembered. Of course, this time I looked at the statue and every detail. The cut of the suit, the shape and size of the hands, the age lines on the face—it was perfect.

I called the real estate developer as soon as I got home and asked for the name of the person who had sculpted the statue.

"His name is Dominguez," he told me. "Jesus Ygnacio Dominguez. He's a professor over at San Diego State."

When I talked to Dominguez, I discovered that he had been an art professor at the university since 1976. He taught classes in figurative sculpture, wood sculpture, basic drawing, and other three-dimensional design. He also had a list of impressive credits. These included a bronze bust of Ray Kroc, the founder of McDonald's Restaurants, which stands at Qualcomm Stadium in San Diego; a relief sculpture at the main library in Fullerton, California; and another sculpture that stands at the entrance to one of the Frank Lloyd Wright houses at Barnsdall Art Park in Los Angeles.

I was also pleased to discover that, in addition to being extremely talented, he was a warm and compassionate man who volunteered at the Braille Institute. He was the type of guy who could understand how much Fred Lebow meant to the City of New York and the world of running.

I asked him if he had ever heard of Fred Lebow and he said he hadn't. I wasn't surprised, because Fred was always content to remain in the background, which was precisely one of the reasons I wanted to honor him with a statue. Most serious marathoners knew who Fred was. People who weren't marathoners didn't.

I asked Dominguez if he knew about the New York City Marathon.

"Of course," he answered. "He has something to do with that?"

"He was one of the co-founders who started it," I answered. "He runs it."

We talked for a while longer, and I could tell that he was impressed by what I had to say. At the same time, I was pleased by what I heard from Professor Dominguez. It didn't take me very long to decide that he was the one I wanted to sculpt Fred's statue.

Professor Dominguez felt the same way. The more he heard about Fred, the more he wanted to be involved. He believed in the project so much that he agreed to sculpt the statue for $35,000, which was among the lowest estimates I had been given. He was also willing to work with me on payment and didn't ask for a huge down payment to get started.

MAKING A MAQUETTE

I didn't know anything about statue making, so Dominguez explained to me that the first step was to make a maquette, a statuette that would be about roughly one-fourth the size of the final life-size statue. (Maquette is French for "scale model.") The maquette also serves as the model for the finished project and allows for tweaks to be made as the sculpture takes shape.

During the course of our conversation, Dominguez and I discovered that we lived within a mile of each other in La Mesa, a suburb of San Diego. That was especially good news because Dominguez planned to do the work in his garage/studio.

I told him that Fred was ill with cancer and I was anxious to get going. There was only one problem: I had to come up with enough money to pay for the materials we needed, which meant an outlay of $2,000. I wasn't exactly sure where the money was coming from, but I didn't want to let on.

"How long will it take you?" I asked.

"When do you need it?"

"November second."

"You mean this year? Seven months from now?"

I told him, "We're planning to honor Fred at a luncheon at the Waldorf Astoria in New York" I explained, "That's two days before the Marathon. Fred will be there—along with many big-name runners, elected city officials, and other celebrities. That's where I want to unveil the maquette statue of Fred."

Dominguez nodded. "I'll get started right away."

"What do you need from me?" I asked.

"The money for the materials."

"Of course."

"And then I need some photographs—portraits, if you can get some. If not, I need the best-quality photos you can get, and I need to see him from all angles."

I wasn't exactly sure how I'd accomplish that since Fred still didn't know about the statue, but I made a note to call Anne Roberts and see what she could do to help.

"What else?" I asked.

"I need to know how big he is. How tall, how much he weighs, his shoe size..."

There were dozens of small details I'd never even thought about. Statue-making is a meticulous business.

"I also need to know what you want the statue to look like. Do you want him to be running? Standing?"

That was easy. I told him I wanted the statue to show Fred the way I had first seen him: looking at his watch. I also explained that I didn't want Fred's facial expression to look like he was impatient. He shouldn't be looking at his watch as if to say, *What took you so long?* but rather, *Come on! You're doing great! You're going to be proud of your time!*

That was the way he made me feel, even though I knew that, at four and a half hours, I certainly wasn't setting any course records.

CARE PACKAGE FROM ANNE

I called Anne Roberts right away and told her I needed her help.

"I need photos of Fred," I said. "If he's had a portrait taken, I need that. If you can find some snapshots, that's good, too. I need head shots, full body shots, whatever you can get your hands on. Oh, and it would also be great if you could get me his weight, his height, and all that sort of thing."

Anne replied that she'd see what she could do, and I could hear the excitement in her voice when I told her about my meeting with Dominguez.

A few days later a box from New York City arrived. I tore into it immediately and was delighted to see that she had done even more than I'd asked. Inside I found a manila envelope with ten or twelve top-quality photos of Fred, plus a well-worn pair of size nine Asics brand running shoes. And there was something else, wrapped in tissue paper. What could this be?

Was it a windbreaker? No, wait. It was more than that. Anne had sent me one of Fred's track suits. I'm still not certain how she managed that—but she did, and it was a tremendous help to me and Jesus Dominguez.

A GENEROUS DONATION

There was still one important matter that needed immediate attention. I still had to come up with the money Dominguez needed to get started—$2,000.

Now I had to phone Ollie one more time. In April, three of us, Allan Steinfeld of the New York Road Runners Club, Inc., J. Oliver Crom, President and CEO of Dale Carnegie, and my company, Mitrovich and Associates, Inc., signed an agreement to host the luncheon in November. The entire financial burden of the luncheon rested on the Dale Carnegie organization, not the New York Road Runners Club (NYRRC) or Mitrovich and Associates.

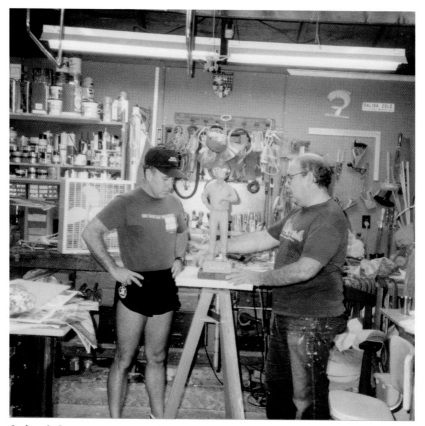

Sculptor's Garage – Dan Mitrovich, Jesus Dominquez

April was only one month after I came up with the idea to do the statue of Fred. But somehow I had never shared this with Ollie. Now I did not have a choice; I needed to share my idea and ask for $2,000.

When I told him what I needed the money to pay for a maquette, he said he would do it; however, he said, "If you get this statue of Fred made, please make certain you get permission to place it in the park, as I do not want it to end up in my backyard."

BIG EVENT—BIGGER ANNOUNCEMENT

"I am delighted to send warm greetings to all those who are gathered for the New York City Marathon Luncheon. The spirit and the purpose of the New York City Marathon have long been exemplified by its founder, Fred Lebow. Simply put, Fred and his fellow race organizers have helped all of us to see that the qualities that are needed to excel in running are also those that are necessary to excel in life. Barbara joins me in sending best wishes for an enjoyable luncheon. God bless you."

—President George H.W. Bush

OVER THE NEXT FEW DAYS, WEEKS, and months, an amazing transformation took place in Jesus Dominguez's garage.

I didn't want to put undue pressure on him, so I tried not to stop by very often. Each time I did I was amazed to see how the miniature version of the statue was taking shape. Dominguez worked for hours to make sure one simple feature was right. Often he saw flaws where I saw perfection.

That hand looked just right to me. But not to the sculptor. He smoothed, massaged, and fussed over every detail. Watching him work made me smile. There was not a doubt in my mind that I had hired the right man.

RUNNING BOSTON

In April, at Fred's invitation, I traveled to Boston and ran in the first of my five Boston Marathons. I finished in 4:09:16, more than half an hour ahead of my time in New York City the previous year, but almost two hours behind the winner, Ibrahim Hussein of Kenya. Hussein was the first Kenyan to win in Boston, but he certainly wasn't the last. His victory began a Kenyan domination that continued for the next two decades.

I love running in Boston. There's so much to see there that you can run for miles and not even know it. Running along Commonwealth Avenue Mall in Back Bay to the Harvard Bridge, crossing over the Charles River on the Harvard Bridge to Cambridge, past the Massachusetts Institute of Technology (MIT), and along the Charles to Longfellow Bridge. Crossing over and through Beacon Hill on Charles Street and through Commonwealth Park and Boston Common.

You can run through the Financial District and over to North End, through Faneuil Hall Marketplace, Quincy Market, and past what was my favorite running store, The Bill Rodgers Running Center. It was run by his brother, Charlie, but closed in 2013. (Now you can shop online at www.billrodgersrunningcenter.com.) You can run the Freedom Trail and pass the *USS Constitution*. And of course one should never run Boston without running around the great Fenway Park. There is just no end in Boston for a great run!

I honestly feel that the New York City and Boston marathons are the two greatest marathons in the world. I'm proud that I've participated in both of them. But, exciting as it is to run in Boston, it is New York that has my heart.

PLANNING THE LUNCHEON

I returned home to find that the maquette version of Fred's statue was slowly nearing perfection. More excited than ever, I turned my attention to the planned luncheon in November in New York City, where Fred would be honored and the plan for the statue in Central Park would be revealed to the general public.

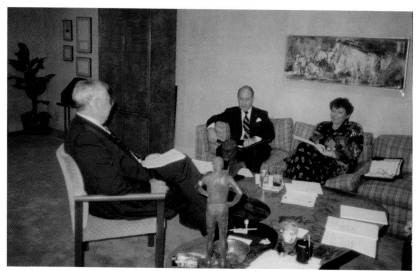

10/31/1991 Dale Carnegie Headquarters, Jericho, Long Island, New York. J. Oliver Crom, Dan Mitrovich, Linda Brannon

Understanding that November was just six months away, I felt it would be necessary to go to New York City and meet with J. Oliver Crom at Dale Carnegie to help plan the event. I asked Linda to travel with me and have some fun in the city.

She agreed to come, but my promise of fun just did not happen, as we were both thrown into a planning session for the luncheon with Dale Carnegie people.

J. Oliver Crom, Peter and Brenda Johnson, Michael Crom, Anne Roberts, Linda Brannon, who I would later marry, and me.

Dale Carnegie and Associates, under the leadership of J. Oliver Crom, not only provided the money we needed to get the maquette done, but also underwrote the tribute luncheon, which was to be held on November 2, 1991, at the Waldorf Astoria in New York City. In addition Dale Carnegie underwrote many of the tables at the luncheon, and Crom made another donation in the amount of $10,000 to Sloan-Kettering Cancer Research as a special favor for Fred.

Our West Coast team 2,812 miles away consisted of me, Linda Brannon, and her staff at Linda Brannon and Associates. She never

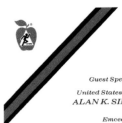

New York City Marathon® Corporate Luncheon

Honoring
FRED LEBOW

Celebrating 22 years of the NYC Marathon

Guest Speaker

United States Senator
ALAN K. SIMPSON

Emcee
GEORGE PLIMPTON

Thursday, October 31, 1991

Starlight Roof, The Waldorf Astoria
New York, New York

Benefitting:

Memorial Sloan-Kettering Cancer Center

Event Sponsor

J. OLIVER CROM

DALE CARNEGIE AND ASSOCIATES

Tables of 10
$2,000.00

Individual Tickets
$225.00

1991 Luncheon Invitation copy

ASK ME ABOUT . . .

New York City Marathon® Tribute Committee

" The Fred Lebow Sculpture "

The Committee

Grete Waitz, Bill Rodgers, Alberto Salazar,
Joan Benoit Samuelson, George Plimpton,
U.S. Senator Allan K. Simpson, J. Olliver Crom,
Allan Steinfeld, Dr. William A. Burke,
Ollan Cassell, Steve Scott, Ron Tabb, David Hall,
and many more . . .

knew what was in store for her or how much she would have to give of her time to help me with the luncheon.

It was a huge undertaking, with no responsibility falling on any of the New York Road Runners Club members. You may recall I only asked for Fred to show up and loan us the official banner of the New York City Marathon.

We all worked hard to get the invitations sent out to some of the biggest names in sports, entertainment, business, and politics.

I was not surprised when the RSVPs came in with positive replies. Almost everyone invited said they were going to be there. Many included notes saying they wouldn't miss it for anything and that they were delighted Fred was going to get some of the recognition he deserved. Nobody knew that I planned to unveil a maquette of Fred or that I would announce there would someday be a life-sized statue of Fred Lebow in Central Park.

MASTER OF CEREMONIES

We were thrilled when Senator Alan Simpson agreed to give the keynote speech. The senator had become a great admirer of Fred when he took him to meet President Bush and was most happy to accept the invitation. That left one spot to fill: Master of Ceremonies.

For this I turned to one of my favorite authors and personalities, the legendary George Plimpton.

Plimpton was a longtime friend of my brother George. George, who truly admired and respected Plimpton, had the privilege of introducing him at a number of public events. Plimpton, seemingly embarrassed by my brother's introductions, began calling my brother "the King of Hyperbole."

My brother once wrote of Plimpton: "He was one of the best storytellers who ever graced a platform, stood behind a podium, or spoke into a microphone." I knew Plimpton would be a great choice for emcee. First of all, he was a New Yorker, and New Yorkers love other New Yorkers! Second, he was a big name who would add to the luster of the luncheon and bring media attention, which could only help our cause.

When I asked Plimpton to serve as emcee, he immediately said yes. Although he didn't personally know Fred Lebow, he knew what the man meant to the City of New York. But when I told him about my plan to honor Fred Lebow with a statue in Central Park, he was incredulous.

"You think you're going to just put up a statue?" he asked. "Do you have any idea how tough that's going to be?"

That was my first inclination that things might not go as easily as I had always thought. Okay, maybe I didn't know the New York City bureaucracy all that well. But Fred was worthy of the honor. Certainly they would support it, I thought.

PREPARATIONS

The luncheon was held in the Starlight Room at the Waldorf Astoria Hotel at noon on Friday, just two days before the twenty-second running of the New York City Marathon. Prior to the luncheon there was so much to do, including going up to the Road Runners Club at 9 E. 89th Street to pick up the official New York City Marathon banner, which would be draped across the finish line on Sunday. Fred was worried about it, as it was the only one they had, yet they were entrusting it to me for the luncheon.

By Friday I had still not picked up the banner, and now it was getting really close to when we needed to be at the hotel. Linda and I got a cab and headed up to the Road Runners Club. We picked up the banner and hailed another cab to take us to the Waldorf, forty-nine blocks back down Park Avenue to 50th Street. We were running way behind in time, and I was telling the New York cabbie to get a move on it. He was not too pleased with me telling him how to drive, and if you've ever been in a New York cab, you'll certainly understand what I am saying.

As we got close to 50th Street and the Waldorf, we hit a huge traffic jam. Now I was getting really nervous, and also, for some reason, I worried that the banner we had just picked up was somehow not in the trunk. So when the cab stopped I jumped out to take a look, and in doing so I opened the door into another cab and caused a little scratch.

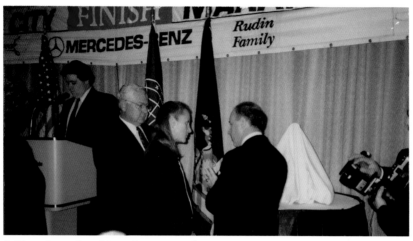

J. Oliver Crom, Grete Waitz, Dan Mitrovich

Of course the banner was in the trunk, and I jumped back in just as our cab was about to move again. The driver of the other cab was eloquently expressing his fury about the scratch, but our cab driver just stepped on it and that was that. You can bet I gave that driver a large tip.

We immediately went up to the Starlight Room of the hotel to take care of pre-luncheon business. Having the hotel staff drape the New York City Marathon banner across the room. Meet with J. Oliver Crom, Senator Simpson, George Plimpton, and Grete Waitz. It was important to go over with Grete how she would handle the unveiling of the Statue of Fred.

I also needed to talk with brother George and Linda about some of the agenda items that were changing on us by the minute.

After meeting with George and Linda, I spent time with Anne Roberts and Carl Lewis, as well as Steve Scott and my dear friend C. Emmett Mahle who flew in from Sacramento, California for the luncheon and Sunday's Marathon.

I hold the greatest of respect for Emmett who was a graduate of West Point, having served and commanded an airborne company in 173 Airborne Brigade in Vietnam in 1970. Emmet's family has a long tradition of serving in the military of our country.

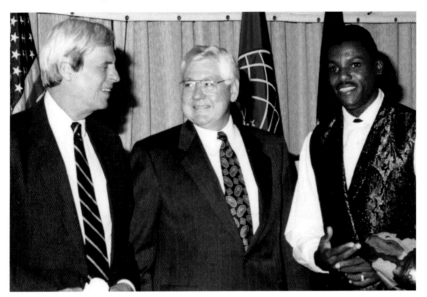

George Plimpton, J. Oliver Crom, Carl Lewis

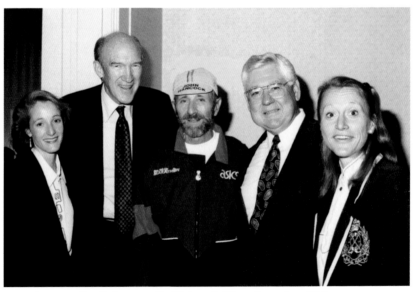

Susan Simpson, Alan K. Simpson, Fred Lebow, J. Oliver Crom, Grete Waitz

Emmet and his wife Barbara's son, Colin Mahle graduated from VMI, class of 2000, has served nine tours in the military. Fifteen months in Korea, four tours in Iraq, and four tours in Afghanistan.

His wife Charlsey who graduated from West Point in 2004 has also served two tours in Iraq.

HUGE SUCCESS

When I saw Fred he looked a little frail to me. Anne told me that he was doing pretty well, his cancer was responding to treatment, and he was starting to regain his strength and stamina. He was his usual talkative self and having a great time. So was everyone else, me included. Of course it is always difficult to enjoy your own event, as the only time you can relax is after everyone has left and it is officially over.

From all accounts, however, the luncheon was a huge success. J. Oliver Crom welcomed everybody in attendance and officially opened the luncheon. It was then my pleasure to introduce a friend of mine,

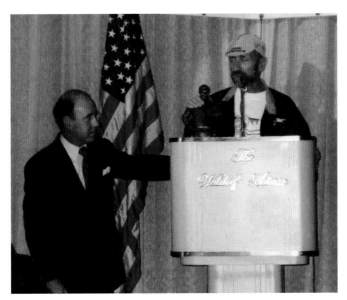

Acceptance of Maquette – Dan Mitrovich, Fred Lebow

Anne Hampton Callaway, to sing a new song, "At the Same Time," for which she had written the lyrics and the music. Her song was later recorded by Barbara Streisand. After Anne's beautiful voice and song set the tone for the luncheon, I asked my brother George to introduce George Plimpton, who, of course, softened the audience up with some of his great humor. Plimpton then introduced Alan K. Simpson. The senator opened by reading a welcoming letter from President Bush and then gave the keynote speech.

We were all so blessed to have such great talent there to honor Fred. There was no other place in New York City on that day that had such notables in attendance.

As we neared the conclusion of the luncheon, Plimpton again made his way to the microphone and asked for everyone's attention.

The loud buzz of conversation quieted to a murmur and then fell silent as Plimpton explained that I had a special announcement to make.

I stepped to the podium and thanked everyone for coming to honor Fred. I then asked those in attendance to turn their attention to the table to my left where Grete Waitz was standing. As people turned their eyes in her direction, Grete took the veil off the maquette statue.

I then invited Fred to join me at the podium. Fred and I held the maquette as I announced that there would someday be a life-sized version

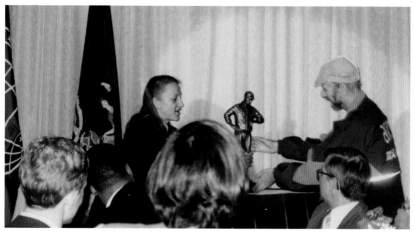

Grete Waitz, Fred Lebow, and Little Fred

68

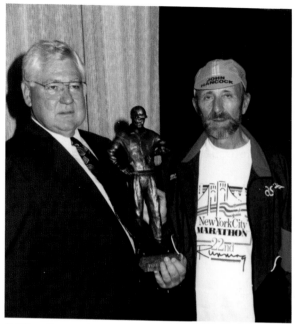

J. Oliver Crom and Fred Lebow

of this statue standing in Central Park to honor Fred for his contribution to the City of New York and runners throughout the world.

Sadly, I later found out from Anne Roberts that Fred didn't really understand. He thought he was being presented with an award and didn't comprehend that a statue was going to be erected in his honor.

On top of that, Linda got a pretty good idea of what we would be facing as she sat with representatives of Mayor Dinkins's office and with Parks Commissioner Henry Stern. They were polite but made it clear to her that putting a statue in New York's Central Park was not likely to happen.

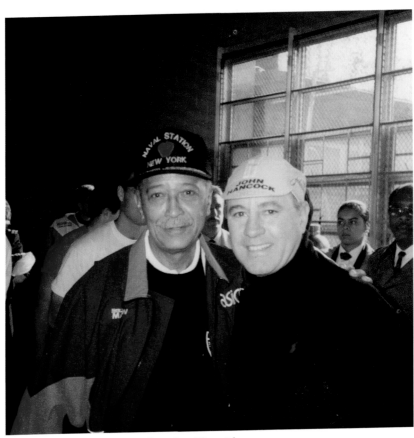

New York City Mayor David Dinkins, Dan Mitrovich

8

NEW YORK, NEW YORK

"You think you're going to just put up a statue? Do you have any idea how tough that's going to be?"

—*George Plimpton*

TWO DAYS AFTER OUR LUNCHEON AT the Waldorf, I ran in the 1991 New York City Marathon.

Anne Roberts arranged for me and my friend Emmett Mahle to be placed on the elite bus carrying runners from Manhattan to the start line. As we got on the bus, we noticed right away there was a huge difference in our bib numbers to the rest of the runners on the bus.

Anne made us sit in the front rows of the bus, but Emmett felt really out of place, as our numbers were so different than the others. Mine was 9821 and Emmett's was 9822. The numbers on the guys seated across form us started with One, Two, and Three. Emmett was so embarrassed he just could not sit there, so he moved all the way to the back. I started to get up to join him, but Anne told me to sit down, as I had earned the privilege to sit up front. Wow, that was really nice, but, like Emmett, I was embarrassed by it!

Linda was already on the bus as she had offered to volunteer and was assigned to be part of the escort team for the elite runners. We had a police escort to Staten Island and the start, which was at the base of the Verrazano Bridge. The bus just behind us, also with a police escort, had an accident going through the Brooklyn-Battery Tunnel: one of the Police motorcycles went down, causing an accident. Some of the runners were actually hurt by the accident and had to withdraw from the race. I should also note that none of the runners filed any lawsuits! I say this, as these days people sue for anything and everything. I like to think that we runners are a special breed of people!

Prior to the cannon being fired to signal the race to begin, Linda was part of the human chain at the start. It was her job, along with about fifty others, to hold back the 40,000-plus runners. Here is what happened, in her own words.

"Never having been to a marathon, let alone the New York City Marathon, I had no idea what to expect when I asked Anne Roberts if I could volunteer. Anne was extremely busy, running in ten directions at once with people everywhere. She looked at me and grabbed a young man, assigned him to take me with him, and told me to stay with him and do what he did.

"We rode the bus out to Staten Island and went with the elite runners to a gymnasium. We were there for a while when my guide told me to lock arms to form a circle and escort the elite runners to the start line. When we got to the start, those in the circle continued to lock arms and form a straight line. The runners pressed hard up against us, and it was really hard to keep them behind the line. You can imagine my shock when I realized where I was and what I was doing, but there was no time to think—the gun went off! It was a stampede!

"I have no idea what happened next, but the angels were certainly with me. I found myself up on a high pilaster (higher than I could climb up or jump down from). From there I watched the sea of runners go by and then they were gone. All was extremely quiet; there was no one in sight. I was there by myself, stuck on a pilaster at the entrance to the Verrazano Bridge, looking down on a road covered in runner's discarded sweats.

"Finally, two knights in shining armor came by in a truck. They had to be surprised to find me. After helping me down, they drove me to my next destination—the finish line—with a police escort, no less."

Linda's next volunteer activity was at the finish line in Central Park as one of the official greeters of the elite finishers. She was told to look for the blue dot on the running bibs; that would signal to her that they were elite runners. Linda thought this would be a good place to be, as she could then welcome me across the finish line. Working the finish line proved to be quite an adventure for Linda, as well. Here is what happened.

"When my rescuers delivered me safe and sound to the finish in Central Park, they told me to go to a tent on a knoll just past the finishing chutes. There I would meet the volunteers I was going to work with and get my instructions.

"I was really excited about having the chance to be right at the finish line, especially because I would be able to be there when Dan finished and could escort him to the tent. Much like the morning, however, I was not prepared for what would happen next.

"I was really looking forward to meeting everyone, but when I walked in the tent, I wasn't especially welcomed. After some stares someone finally asked me, "Who are you and how did you get here?" The volunteers were a pretty close-knit group and Never-Been-to-a-Marathon-Before-Linda clearly did not belong. Once I told them that I was there with Dan Mitrovich—who was going to put a statue of Fred in Central Park—all that changed. I was welcomed and had an incredibly wonderful afternoon at the finish line. It brings tears to my eyes as I write this. To be at the finish line is an incredible once-in-a-lifetime opportunity that I will never forget.

"The first thing I learned is how amazing and dedicated New York Marathon volunteers are. There are, on average, 12,000 volunteers. Most of them come back every year, and many love it so much they schedule their vacations around the marathon. They work their way into volunteer positions. Being allowed to work the finish line is one of the most sought-after positions. It is because of the thousands of volunteers that the marathon has excellent crowd control and flows so smoothly.

"My job, as Dan said, was to look for the blue dot on running bibs and escort those with the blue dot up to the tent. Being in the chutes, looking for the blue dots on runners' bibs, was absolutely magical. I was surrounded by the pure joy of the runners as they crossed the finish line. Many got down on their knees and kissed the ground, others jumped for joy, some cried, all celebrated. As for me, that day I had the privilege of being hugged, kissed, high fived, danced with, showered in laughter and with tears by a few thousand runners—men and women—speaking many different languages. I was covered in sweat, dirt, blood, mud, and very happy when Dan crossed the line and we walked up to the tent together.

"I was truly blessed by this experience in so many ways—in the morning by being lifted up out of the way and in the afternoon being surrounded by joy and happiness. I am forever grateful to Dan for wanting to honor Fred, and to Anne for sending me to the start and finish, and to all the volunteers who welcomed me in and guided me throughout the day."

6 MINUTES 13 SECONDS FASTER

Despite not doing as well as I wanted, my time was 6 minutes and 13 seconds better than my 1990 time. I was still exhilarated by the race. The excitement had not diminished at all. The pageantry and grandeur of the occasion confirmed to me what I already knew: the New York City Marathon is, indeed, one of the world's greatest events of any kind.

Coming across the finish line and having Linda greet me was very special to me. She escorted me over to a VIP tent near the finish line. Being able to walk just about seventy-five yards was certainly a lot better than the year before when I had to walk a mile to the truck that carried our runners' running bags. Being able to get inside a tent and out of the cold was very special. As most of us runners know, we are very vulnerable to temperature at the end of a race.

Unfortunately, I never saw my friend Emmet again after the race, as somehow he ended up somewhere else and nowhere around me and Linda.

The evening after the race Linda and I joined a partner of mine, Seymour Heller, for dinner at one of his favorite Italian restaurants.

The next day we flew home to California. But the huge effort to get ready for the luncheon three days before was starting to sink in. Making the announcement about the life-size statue of Fred that would be placed in New York's Central Park was now a reality, and now I would have to actually try to make it happen.

It had taken a huge effort on our part to have the maquette ready for unveiling at the luncheon, and now I had to think about making a life-size statue. Wow! What do I do next?

HOW TOUGH CAN IT BE?

"It will be easier for a camel to go through the eye of a needle than to put a new statue in Central Park."

—Henry Stern, New York City Parks Commissioner

CITY OF NEW YORK PARKS AND RECREATION

MY FRIEND GEORGE PLIMPTON STILL WASN'T convinced the Fred Lebow statue would ever be standing in New York's Central Park. Of course he was having some good-natured fun at my expense, watching his friend from southern California trying to learn how to navigate through the complex labyrinth of New York City rules and regulations. And he was right to tell me; at the time of the announcement, I really had no idea what it would really mean to fulfill my promise or how it would impact my life over the next ten years.

Despite what I'd heard from George Plimpton and a few other people, I thought I could handle whatever they threw at me, and I felt it was such a worthy, unselfish and much-deserved goal that tens of thousands would rise to assist me. I couldn't have been more wrong.

STATUE MORATORIUM

The first thing I discovered, in a meeting with a mid-level manager at the Parks Department, was that a person had to be dead for seven years before he or she could even be considered for a statue in any New York City park.

"But surely you can make an exception for a man like Fred Lebow," I said.

The man was sympathetic but firm, "No exceptions," he said.

Oh, wait. There was another problem.

No more statues in Central Park. Of any kind. A moratorium had been declared.

Yes, there were dozens of statues in the park. Statues of political leaders, military heroes, authors, actors, and even fictional characters. There were not any statues of sports figures unless, as George Plimpton said, "You consider Balto, the sled dog who saved Alaska's children from a diphtheria epidemic by delivering medicine, a sports figure." There were also no statues of women, with the exception of two fictional characters: one being Alice in Wonderland and the other, at the Bethesda Fountain, being a female winged angel.

It was also becoming increasingly apparent to me that Linda and I could not do this on our own. Many seemed to regard us as outsiders who had no business trying to tell the people of New York what to do. And, of course, we needed to raise money. We needed some big names behind us. More importantly, we needed a name that meant something.

By 1994 I had added to my team a lot of names of power, both within and out of the running community. I added many city, state, and federal officials to the effort—as well as many of the biggest names in running—and it seemed certain that it was only a matter of time until my dream became a reality.

PERMISSION TO USE NAME

I telephoned Fred to get permission to use the name of the New York City Marathon. He never hesitated a bit in giving me permission to use the name.

TRIBUTE COMMITTEE

When Allan Steinfeld signed the letter authorizing the use of the New York City Marathon name, our next move was to formalize our tribute committee into a 501(c)(3).

For this I called my friend Paul Dostart, an attorney and CPA, who had a successful firm, Monroe and Dostart, in San Diego. This was the birth of the New York City Marathon Tribute Committee (NYCMTC).

I formed the New York City Marathon Tribute Committee—rather than the Fred Lebow Tribute Committee—for a very important reason. First, because Fred was not the sort of guy who liked to be in the limelight, and second, because I couldn't be sure that everyone I wanted to talk to would know who he was. Of course almost everyone associated with running would know him, but I wanted to enlist the support of some other celebrities and political leaders who might not have heard of Fred but certainly knew about the New York City Marathon.

SITTING ACROSS FROM HENRY STERN

My next move was to meet with Parks Commissioner Henry J. Stern. I telephoned Mr. Stern to set a meeting in his office at the Arsenal at Fifth Avenue and 64th Street, the headquarters of the New York City Parks Department. Stern ran a department with more than 4,000 employees and a $200 million annual budget, but he took pride in being a hands-on manager. He was also a very smart man, having graduated from Harvard Law School at age twenty-two. He worked very hard to keep up with everything that happened on his watch.

Stern was responsible for overseeing more than 28,000 acres of parks in New York City that include 980 playgrounds, 614 ball fields, thirty-five recreation centers and fourteen miles of beaches. Part of those acres include Central Park, consisting of 843 acres. It is 2.5 miles long between 59th Street and 110th Street and is one-half mile across between Fifth Avenue and Central Park West (CPW).

Mayor Ed Koch told *New York* magazine's Joe Klein, "Henry knows more about the city than anyone. He knows everything that's happened since Peter Minuet." Minuet, as you may recall, was the Dutchman who allegedly gave the Indians $24 worth of beads and trinkets for Manhattan Island.

Stern had a reputation for working long, hard hours, seven days a week. On Saturdays and Sundays, when the city's 1,000-plus parks were filled to near capacity, he often made the rounds to ensure those parks were meeting the needs of New York's seven million-plus residents.

I quickly discovered that Stern was tough.

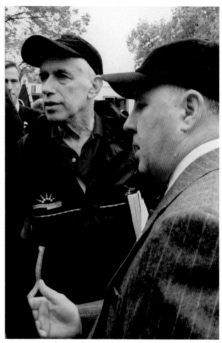

Commissioner of City of New York Parks and Recreation – Henry Stern, Dan Mitrovich

"There's no way this is going to happen," he told me, speaking in a tone that made me think he must get requests for new statues all the time.

As a matter of fact, he did.

And he turned them all down, no matter what he thought about the worthiness of the idea.

Stern, an avid swimmer, had high regard for Fred Lebow. He says now, "The Marathon meant a lot for New York City. It brought in thousands of runners, who spent millions of dollars. And I appreciated the fact that Fred Lebow got so many people into running, which is such a healthy thing to do."

But none of that mattered when it came to opening a spot for Fred's statue in Central Park.

"Let me put it this way," he said with a chuckle. "It will be easier for a camel to go through the eye of a needle than to put a statue in Central

Park." He added, "The park was really becoming overcrowded. We get tons of requests for statues—way too many to consider."

Stern was sympathetic, but unyielding.

I didn't know it at the time, but in the early 1980s more than 250,000 people had signed petitions asking the city to lift the moratorium so a life-size statue of John Lennon could be placed in the park. But today, although there is an area of the park dedicated to Lennon, there is no statue there. If a worldwide hero like John Lennon couldn't make it into the park, what chance did Fred Lebow have?

Still, I knew that Fred Lebow had earned his place, and I wasn't about to give up just because of a few rejections and a moratorium. I promised Stern that I'd be back in touch, and I kept my promise.

When I asked him if he remembers all those meetings, he says, "You were awfully persistent, but you had to be. If you have a vision, you have to keep pushing forward. I didn't mind that you were a *nudje*. (*Nudje* is Hebrew word that best translates as "bother" or "pest.") You had something you wanted to do, you were determined. I couldn't be put off by that. Truth is, I was interested in this right from the beginning. I knew Fred, and I felt he was worthy of such an honor."

Sometimes, in my dealing with Henry Stern and the rest of the New York City Parks Department, I felt like I was banging my head against an unyielding wall. But I was motivated by Fred Lebow's unique character, as well as his contributions to the city, the world of running, and unity between diverse cultures. I saw how the Marathon he started had brought together people from every one of New York's five boroughs. Whites, Blacks, Hispanics, Italians, Orthodox Jews, Asians. I also saw how the Marathon brought together people from almost every country and culture around the world.

If anyone in our day deserved to be added to the roster of heroes in Central Park, surely Fred Lebow did.

I knew I was going to have to put in a great deal of hard work to make it happen, but I was ready to roll up my sleeves and do whatever it took. I expected opposition. But I also expected that I could and would overcome it.

GATHERING SUPPORT

I learned a long time ago that you can't get upset if people don't call you back. You can't get angry if they won't take the time to talk to you or if they tell you that you're calling at a bad time. Whenever someone tells me something like that, I say, politely, "Fine. I understand. I'll call you another time." Then I quickly get off the phone and make a note to follow up. I don't keep them hanging on the phone, which could make them so aggravated they'll never talk to me at all. I've learned that people will eventually talk to you, but you have to get them at a time when it's good for them to talk.

Will Rogers famously said that he never met a man he didn't like. I have a feeling he knew how important it is to find the right time to talk to people. Because if you do that, you'll find that there are very few truly unfriendly or uncooperative people in the world.

I've had people tell me about a celebrity, "Oh, I don't like that person." When I ask why, they tell me, "Well, I met him, and he was rude."

That brings up a few more questions: Did you catch him or her on a bad day? Did you just walk up to the person, interrupt what they were doing, and launch into a conversation about yourself? Was he rude because you were rude first?"

I may not always succeed, and if I don't, I try not to let it get to me. If it does, I look for constructive ways to deal with it—like running.

I did an awful lot of running during those days as I struggled to deal with the bureaucracy and untangle the red tape of America's largest city.

THE COMMITTEE OF TWENTY-THREE

"If you want to win a Super Bowl, a World Series, an NBA title, an Oscar, a Tony Award, or place a statue in New York's Central Park, you need to assemble the best team you can. My team of twenty-three were indeed the best!"

—Daniel S. Mitrovich

THE LUNCHEON COMMITTEE WAS POWERFUL IN its own right, but now I wanted to expand that power in forming the New York City Marathon Tribute Committee.

I started by asking those who served on the original luncheon committee to continue with the now formalized New York City Marathon Tribute Committee. I received a strong yes from all. By now they knew exactly what I had promised, and they all knew it would not be easy, but for Fred they went along anyway!

This strong, courageous man, Fred Lebow, had empowered so many people all over the world. But, like all of us, sometimes he needed a little help from his friends. Billy Rodgers and Grete Waitz, for example, were both tremendously important to Fred in the development of the New York City Marathon, and now they were once again doing their part for Fred and my goal to place a statue of him in Central Park.

I needed to have at least four people on the board of directors, and for that I choose two members who lived close to me in California; it may be important to obtain their signatures from time to time, and this made it much easier. I also wanted to have Anne Roberts on that board. She had played such an important part in helping me all along the way, she was the closest to Fred, and she was part of the New York Road Runners Club.

So the board of directors of the New York City Marathon Tribute Committee consisted of Steve Scott, Keith Jeffers, Anne Roberts, and me.

The Committee Chairman was J. Oliver Crom, and Honorary Chairs were Senator Alan K. Simpson, Grete Waitz, and Bill Rodgers.

INTRODUCTION OF THE COMMITTEE

BILL RODGERS

Rodgers won four straight New York City Marathons: 1976 (2:10:10), 1977 (2:11:28), 1978 (2:12:12), and 1979 (2:11:42). He also won the Boston Marathon four times: 1975 (2:09:55), 1978 (2:10:13), 1979 (2:09:27), and 1980 (2:12:11). It is a shame—as it was for all the athletes—that he didn't get to participate in the 1980 Olympics in the Soviet Union due to the US boycott. There is no doubt in my mind that Billy most likely would have won the Olympic Gold, as he was in top form in 1980. Rodgers ran fifty-nine marathons during his career, including one at the 1976 Olympics, and completed twenty-eight of them in less than 2:15.

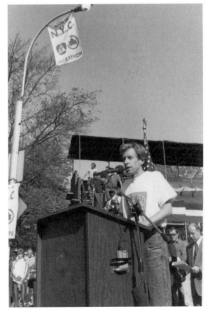

Bill Rodgers

I remember asking him a question one day. "Bill, in all your marathon runs, did you ever want to just drop out of the race and quit?" I told him that in every one of my five Boston Marathons, at about the five-mile mark out from Hopkinton on Union Street in Ashland, there was, and is still, a Dunkin' Donuts shop. And in each of those races, I would just look over there, and my mind would say, *Stop running, go get a donut and a hot cup of coffee, take a seat, and just watch all those runners go on by*.

He told me that there was never a race that the thought of stopping did not come to mind. With that, he made me feel normal.

He also told me something else. "You know, I have so much respect for you runners who are out there for such a long period of time." He said, "Dan, you are out there almost four hours and I am only out there for just a little over two. I can't imagine running for that long of time!"

Even though Rodgers had such a great record in New York, things didn't start out so well for him there. In talking with Anne Roberts, she told me a story. In 1976, after celebrating the first of his four consecutive victories, Rodgers couldn't find his car.

Had it been stolen? No.

It turned out that his Volkswagen had been towed away for being illegally parked, and it would cost $100 to get the car out of storage. Although there was very little prize money for winners in those days, Fred gave him the $100 he needed to get his car back.

Rodgers always thought the New York City Marathon should pay big money to get top-name runners, but Fred didn't believe it was necessary. After all, he wondered, why should he pay people who were going to get tons of publicity for running in the world's biggest and best marathon?

Over the years Bill Rodgers eventually became one of Lebow's closest friends, and he accepted without hesitation when he was asked to serve as an honorary chairman of the Tribute Committee.

GRETE THE GREAT

As much as Bill Rodgers meant to the New York City Marathon, Waitz meant even more. The exceptional runner from Norway won the Women's Division of the New York City Marathon an incredible nine times.

This wonderful woman from Oslo was one of the nicest people you could ever meet. I feel truly treasured and blessed that I had that great pleasure to be able to call her a friend. For me it's hard to comprehend how she did all those marathons in New York. Her wins were all in a span of eleven years, and she didn't run in the '81 or '87 New York City Marathons. I do not ever see anyone, man or woman, doing what she did again in my or anyone else's lifetime!

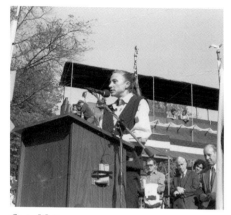
Grete Waitz

She first ran in New York in 1978 after Fred issued a personal invitation to her. She not only won the race, she set a new record time of 2:32:30, taking two full minutes off the women's world record. She broke her own record in 1979 in a time of 2:27:33, 1980 (2:25:41), 1982 (2:27:14), 1983 (2:27:00), 1984 (2:29:30), 1985 (2:28:34), 1986 (2:28:06), 1988 (2:28:07), and 1990 (2:34:34).

Grete lowered the women's world marathon time by nine minutes, setting that time in the London Marathon in 1983.

She won the Stockholm Marathon in 2:28:24, was victorious at the 1983 World Championships in Helsinki, and captured a silver medal at the 1984 Olympics in Los Angeles.

In addition to her marathon victories, she was a five-time World Cross Country Champion.

Her success was particularly gratifying to Fred, who had sought from the very beginning to open up marathoning to women. Waitz shared that joy and that belief, and she and Fred became great friends. She told author Ron Rubin, "He visited me in Oslo many times, and sometimes for no particular reason. Every time I went to New York, I went to the club to see him. He would call me in Norway just to ask how I was doing or how [my husband] Jack was doing."

She also said, "All major cities in the world have a marathon and Fred started it all. He's the inspiration to every race organizer."

Fred replied, "I've always said that if a computer could put together an ideal runner, it would be Grete. She's the Queen of the Road, but she doesn't behave like a monarch. She's a very nice person."

When I asked her to serve on the New York City Marathon Tribute Committee, like Bill Rodgers she immediately said yes. So did a number of other remarkable athletes and leaders from various walks of life. Other members of the Committee included:

ALBERTO SALAZAR

Alberto Salazar, the great marathoner, who was rated number one in the world after he won in both Boston and New York in 1980. Alberto was there the day we unveiled the statue of Fred. He came to the podium and said some wonderful things about his personal friend Fred Lebow. Salazar was born in Cuba in 1958 and then moved with his family to America.

He went to High School in Wayland, Massachusetts. He was the state cross country champion in 1975 and became a member of the Boston

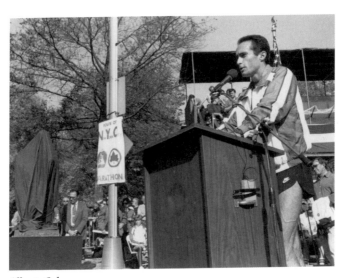

Alberto Salazar

Track Club. After high school he went to the University of Oregon, graduating in 1981 after winning All-American honors.

Salazar said he felt like Fred was a member of his family and added that Lebow was the only race director who made it a point to keep in touch with him after he retired from competitive running. Ten years after Salazar's last race, he was still in touch with Fred, which is more evidence that Fred cared about his runners as people and not just as athletes.

Alberto won three consecutive New York City Marathons: 1980, with a time of 2:09:41, 1981 (2:08:13), and 1982 (2:09:29).

He also won the Boston Marathon in 1982 with a time of 2:09:29.

He currently coaches and has worked with several American distance runners.

JOAN BENOIT SAMUELSON

I will never forget when I first phoned her in 1991 to ask if she would be on the Luncheon Tribute Committee. She said yes right away, but when I asked her to join us at the luncheon to unveil the maquette of Fred, she said she would not be able to attend. She was going trick-or-treating with her children, Abby and Anders, and that was something very special to her. I was so impressed by her telling me that she could not be there. She certainly had her priorities in the right place!

In 2011, twenty-one years after that phone call, she ran the Boston Marathon with her daughter, Abby, finishing in 2:51:29. Her daughter, Abby, who was running her first Boston, finished in 3:30:36.

"Boston is a special race for me," Samuelson said before the race. "The crowds know and appreciate the athletes competing and their accomplishments, and they never disappoint with their encouragement and excitement on Patriots' Day." (Boston CBS)

I didn't get the chance to meet Joan in person until the unveiling of the Fred Lebow statue on November 4, 1994. The instant I first met her I was a fan, although, from just our phone conversation, I knew I would like her way back in 1991.

Joan was born in Cape Elizabeth, Maine. Today she is a writer, having written such books as *Running Tide* and *Running for Women*.

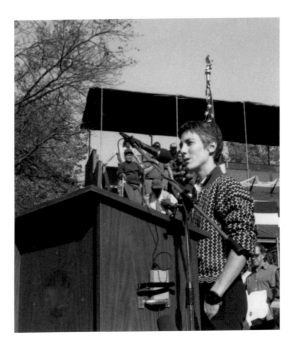

Joan Benoit Samuelson

Her running records are incredible. I became aware of her, along with the rest of the world, when she won a gold medal in the 1984 Olympic Games in Los Angeles. But she also won gold in the 1983 Pan American games. She won the Boston Marathon in 1979 (2:35:15) and again in 1983, setting a world record (2:22:43). And her 1985 Chicago Marathon record time of 2:21:21 stood for 18 years.

GEORGE PLIMPTON

George Plimpton, an American journalist, writer, literary editor, actor and sportsman. The talented best-selling author of sports books like *Paper Lion, Out of My League, The Bogey Man* and more. He founded the *Paris Review* along with Peter Matthiessen and Harold L. Humes. That highly esteemed literary magazine is still being published today. Even after the passing of the three founders, the tradition continues.

George was a great writer and a true gentleman. He appreciated what Fred Lebow had done for the City of New York, although as far as I know, he had only one experience with a marathon, himself. That came when he was a student at Harvard, late in the 1940s. What happened was that Plimpton was trying for a staff writing position on the *Harvard Lampoon*. He was told that, in order to be considered for a position on the magazine, he had to run in the Boston Marathon. But as George told me, "Nobody said I had to run the whole race." So he staked out a spot about two hundred yards from the finish line and waited for the leader to pass. Then he ran out of his hiding spot and sprinted the rest of the way home.

Plimpton found out later that the guy who won the marathon that year nearly had a heart attack when he heard Plimpton's footsteps behind him. He'd thought he had a huge lead—and he did—but Plimpton's stunt made him think he was about to be overtaken. Later on, when he found out what had really happened, he wasn't happy about it. But unlike the infamous Rosie Ruiz, Plimpton never meant to fool anyone.

George would jump on his bike and peddle from his residence at 541 E. 72nd Street to emcee our events for the statue at the Tavern on the Green. It was always fun to watch him peddle up to us.

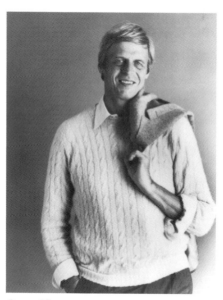

George Plimpton

To know George Plimpton was something very special. I had the privilege of representing him on several speaking engagements over the years, including the Kick-Off Luncheon for the 1989 Super Bowl in Miami. But one of the most fascinating was when my brother George asked me to take George Plimpton to the private residence in La Jolla, California, of Dr. Jonas Salk, the man who discovered the first inactivated polio vaccine. George Plimpton, at the request of *Esquire* magazine, was to determine what Christmas gift to give him the next year. The amount I recall was a gift somewhere up to $10,000. This was an annual thing that *Esquire* magazine would do with ten famous people, and Dr. Salk was one of the ten. I took George into the Salk residence, waited for a few minutes, and decided I would leave them alone. The interview, which he intended to last a couple of hours, had, in fact, lasted but thirty minutes, and Plimpton wanted to leave, as he had one of the most "disillusioning experiences of his life."

Plimpton was unique. I am so fortunate that I had the great pleasure of knowing him and that he agreed to help serve on the committee. When George Plimpton passed away on September 25, 2003, it was a sad day for my brother and me, as it was for so many of his friends. It was a great loss to us all.

He gave the New York City Marathon Tribute Committee a touch of greatness.

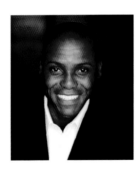

CARL LEWIS

Carl Lewis, the superstar sprinter and long-jumper who won an amazing ten Olympic Medals, nine of them gold. Lewis was chosen as "Sportsman of the Century" by the International Olympic Committee and was named "Olympian of the Century" by *Sports Illustrated*. He was a great admirer of Fred Lebow, as well as a good friend of his.

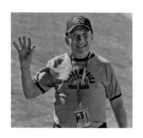

JOE DOUGLAS

Joe Douglas, who founded California's Santa Monica Track Club in 1972. He has coached hundreds of record-setting athletes, including Carl Lewis, Leroy Burrell, Danny Everett, Steve Lewis, Johnny Gray, and Jenny Spangler. Once again, people like Joe Douglas allowed me to include them in the Tribute Committee because it was something for Fred. It certainly had nothing to do with me.

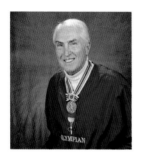

OLLAN CASSELL

Ollan Cassell, the great sprinter who became executive director of the Amateur Athletic Union and president of the Indiana Olympian Association after hanging up his running shoes. In the 1950s and 1960s, Cassell was one of America's best-known runners and won a gold medal in the 1964 Olympics in Tokyo.

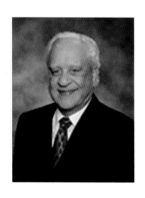

DR. WILLIAM A. BURKE

Dr. William A. Burke, a noted philanthropist who co-founded the Los Angeles Marathon in 1986 and served as that event's president for many years. Dr. Burke, who also served as Commissioner of Tennis for the 1984 Olympic Games in Los Angeles, is married to Dr. Yvonne Brathwaite Burke, the first African-American woman to represent California in Congress.

The great love Bill had for Fred helped me so much in my quest to get the statue in Central Park. Bill became my friend through all of this. I occasionally see him here in Los Angeles, and for a while we were neighbors just a few hundred yards apart in Mandeville Canyon.

Bill stepped up to the plate on several occasions to help me with my cause for Fred. He never said no.

STEVE SCOTT

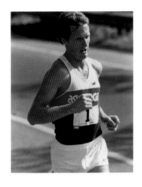

Steve Scott, who ran 136 sub-four-minute miles in his career—an astounding feat, especially considering that many "experts" once insisted that the four-minute barrier could never be broken. England's Roger Bannister shocked the world when he first broke that barrier in 1954. Scott held the American outdoor mile record for more than twenty-six years and was ranked as the number-one miler in the United States on ten separate occasions by *Track & Field News*.

Steve, like so many who said yes to me, were personal friends of Fred and wanted to help in any way they could. I asked Steve to be one of four to serve on the board of directors of our Tribute Committee. Today, Steve is a cross country coach at California State University San Marcos in San Marcos, California.

J. OLIVER CROM

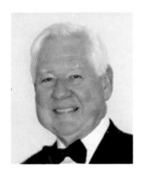

J. Oliver Crom, President and CEO of Dale Carnegie & Associates. Without Oliver's vision and belief in my dream, this project may never have gotten off the ground.

Oliver really does live his life in accordance with the principles of the late Dale Carnegie, author of one of the best books ever written,

How to Win Friends and Influence People. Mr. Carnegie's son-in-law, Oliver, was a great leader for the Dale Carnegie organization for more than forty years.

Oliver is the co-author with his son, Michael A. Crom, of *The Sales Advantage: How to Get it, Keep it, and Sell More Than Ever*.

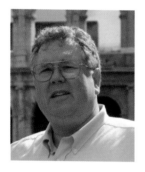

MICHAEL A. CROM

Michael A. Crom, grandson of Dale Carnegie. In addition to being co-author of *The Sales Advantage*, he also co-authored *The Leader in You: How to Win Friends, Influence People, and Succeed in a Changing World*. Michael was the very first person I phoned for help with this huge idea of mine.

It was Michael who talked to his father and then had me make my phone call to him. Michael was my best man when Linda and I married. Years before that, Michael honored me by asking me to serve as godfather to his daughter Nicole.

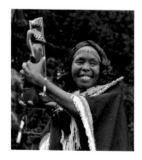

TEGLA LOROUPE

Tegla Loroupe, an accomplished runner from Kenya. Tegla is like a daughter to Anne Roberts. In 1994 she became the first African woman to win the New York City Marathon. She repeated the feat the following year and then finished third in 1998. Loroupe's victory in 1994 made her a hero to thousands of people—especially women—in Kenya and throughout Africa. Sadly for her, Tegla couldn't get any multi-million-dollar endorsement deals from shoe companies because she usually ran barefoot—saving her running shoes for races that she considered particularly tough.

Tegla is one of the greatest female runners of all time, having won marathons and half-marathons all over the world. But I admire her even more for her outspoken support of women's rights, education, and peace. Her Tegla Loroupe Peace Foundation has been instrumental in helping to end hostilities between once-warring tribes in Kenya, Uganda, and Sudan.

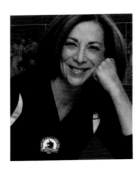

KATHRINE SWITZER

Kathrine Switzer, an American author, television commentator, and marathon runner. She really stood up for what I wanted to do. She told the people of New York that the statue of Fred should be in Central Park and she was shocked by the lack of support I was getting from the City of New York. She went on the air to publicize the statue and to ask people to help me. I cannot say enough good things about her. I am so grateful for her strength and willingness to stand up for Fred.

She was the first woman to run the Boston Marathon as a numbered entry (261). She's rightly famous for taking that brave step in 1967, to be the first and to go against all the power of the Boston Marathon. Jock Semple, the marathon's race director, yelled at her, "Get the hell out of my race and give me those numbers," (referring to her running bib numbers), and then he literally tried to shove her out of "his race!" She went on to finish that race and was the first woman to do so. Boston did not officially allow women in their race until 1972. Switzer went on to win the New York City Marathon in 1974 with a time of 3:07:29. Fifty years later, in 2017, Kathrine, at age seventy, finished the Boston Marathon in a time of 4:44:31 with an average mile of 10:51.

In Kathrine's book, *Marathon Woman* (Carroll & Graf) 2007, she shares her inspiring story and vow to change women's running forever. "And did she! After running thirty-five marathons and creating a global circuit of races for over a million women that led to the inclusion of the women's marathon in the Olympic Games changing forever people's attitudes about women's so-called limitation."

The daughter of a major in the United States Army, she was born in Amberg, Germany, grew up in Fairfax, Virginia, and earned a bachelor's degree in 1968 from Syracuse University. Find more about Kathrine Switzer at info@marathonwoman.com.

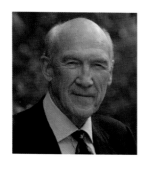

ALAN K. SIMPSON

Alan K. Simpson, former United States Senator from Wyoming (1979 through 1997), Minority Whip of the Senate, and the man who opened the door to the Oval Office so that Fred Lebow could be honored by President George Herbert Walker Bush.

Simpson's father, Milward L. Simpson, served in the U.S. Senate from 1962 to 1967 and served as Governor of Wyoming from 1955 to 1959. Milward was a close personal friend of President George H.W. Bush's father, Prescott Bush, who served as U.S. Senator from Connecticut from 1952 to 1963.

I met Alan Simpson through his great friend, my brother George. Since then he's become my friend, as well, and a friend to my family. By allowing us to use his name, and by being the official speaker at our kick-off luncheon on that October day in 1991, he gave us huge respect that we so needed at that time.

He and his wife, Ann, donated $1,000 to the Tribute Committee. But he also gave of his courage, his intellect, and his goodness—and for that, our Committee shall forever be indebted to Alan K. Simpson!

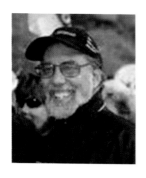

ALLAN STEINFELD

Allan Steinfeld, former President of the New York Road Runners Club, Race Director of the New York City Marathon, Race Director of Fifth Avenue Mile, and Meet Director of the New York Games from 1985 to 1995. Allan was also Fred Lebow's personal friend. He succeeded Fred after Fred's death in 1994.

Steinfeld earned his master's degree in electrical engineering and radio astronomy from Cornell University in 1971, following a bachelor's degree from City College of New York in 1969. That scientific mind, combined with his interest in running, helped make him one of the nation's leading authorities on the technical aspects of road racing.

Both he and his wife, Alice, were major parts of the running of the New York City Marathon. It was Allan whom I communicated with most at the Road Runners Club, and it was Allan who, like me, believed that what Linda and I were doing was worth every bit of the energy it took.

Whenever I called Allan, he made the time to hear me and to assist me.

When I received the call from President Clinton's office inviting me for a private run with the President so I could present to him the first replica of the Fred Lebow statue, I was asked whether I'd want anyone else to join us on this private jog. I told them that Allan Steinfeld and George Hirsch should be part of that special day with President Clinton.

After that incredible run with the President of the United States, Allan, Linda, and I made a trip to Capitol Hill to present two more limited replicas of the statue: one to Alan Simpson and one to Congressman Jose Serrano.

And in 1996 both Allan and Alice joined Linda and me for President Clinton's second inauguration.

Allan, Linda, and I spent a lot of time together. He was a great friend. It was with great sadness we lost him on January 24, 2017. A week later, the New York Road Runners held a special evening in Allan's honor to celebrate his life. He will be missed by all of us that knew him.

GEORGE HIRSCH

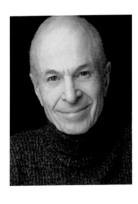

George Hirsch has the power of the pen. He is currently the Chairman of the Board of Directors of The New York Road Runners Club. When I had my idea to honor Fred with a statue, George agreed to serve on the committee. George is founding publisher of *Runners World*, one of the leading running magazines in the world. He graduated from Princeton

University and Harvard Business School. He served in the U.S. Navy as an officer from 1957 to 1960. George helped Fred start the five-borough race in 1976. George is also a great runner. He's run in forty marathons, with a personal best of 2:38, which he did in Boston in 1979 at age forty-four, running much of the race with Joan Benoit. He also joined me, Allan Steinfeld, and my wife, Linda, on our run at the White House with President Clinton in 1995.

George has always been helpful to me in the long quest to place Fred's statue in Central Park. In 2009 he ran his last New York City Marathon at the age of seventy-five with a time of 4:06, but just before that he ran Chicago in 3:58.

I told him that he's my personal hero!

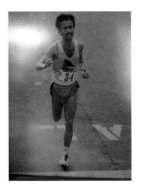

RON TABB

Ron Tabb lived in San Diego when I came up with this idea to honor Fred. Dr. Keith Jeffers told me that Ron would want to be part of this, as he thought so many good things about Fred.

Ron is a former long distance runner, winning the Paris Marathon in 1981 and the Beijing Marathon in 1983. He competed in the 1983 World Championships in Athletics in 1983, finishing eighteenth overall. Ron placed second in the 1983 Boston Marathon behind Greg Meyer (2:09:00), finishing in 2:09:31, which at that time was the fifth-fastest marathon time in U.S. history.

He attended Central Missouri State University and was inducted into their Hall of Fame in 2004. Ron qualified for the 1980 Moscow Olympics, becoming one of the many athletes who suffered due to the Olympic boycott.

DR. KEITH JEFFERS

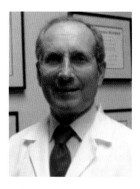

Dr. Keith Jeffers, chiropractor in San Diego, California, known as The Running Doctor. Keith was one of the first people I talked to about my plan. We were both members of the La Jolla Golden Triangle Rotary Club, where I served as President in 1989-1990. Knowing how much he was respected by many great runners, such as Steve Scott and Ron Tabb, I asked Keith to serve on the Committee.

In 1987 he served as President of the San Diego Track Club, an organization to which I also belonged. In 1968 he set the national 10K record with a 33:09 time, beating the old record by two minutes. He won the 1971 San Luis Obispo Marathon, the 1977 Santa Barbara Half-Marathon, the 1981 San Jose, California, Half-Marathon, and ran a 2:38 Boston Marathon in 1983. He won two National Championships as part of the San Diego Track Club. In 1989 he won the Gold Medal in Eugene, Oregon, as a member of the U.S. cross country team. He also placed tenth in the world in the steeplechase. Keith graduated from the University of Santa Barbara with a B.A. in Exercise Physiology.

LINDA MITROVICH

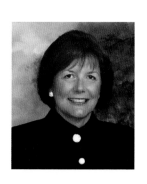

Linda Mitrovich, my wife and partner. After the trip we took to New York in 1991 to meet with the Dale Carnegie people and begin planning that October's luncheon to honor Fred, she never had time to look back.

Asking her to join me on that trip was one of the best invitations I've ever made. She loved Fred Lebow and said she would help in any way possible. I immediately drafted her and her company into the work. The work would take over our lives for the next ten years. Neither of us could possibly have imagined then what her saying yes to me would mean.

Linda served as a City Councilmember and Deputy Mayor in Poway, California. She had graduated from Whittier College, home of Richard Nixon, and later served as a member of the Board of Trustees for the college.

She was honored by the California State Assembly in 1988, as well as by the California State Senate in 1991, as "Woman of the Year." She is president of our company, Solution Strategies International, Inc. For twenty-four years she has played a significant role in helping to create successful strategies for local, state, federal, and international companies.

I know for certain that our committee never could have succeeded in getting Fred "Forever at the Finish Line" without her talents and loving, constant support.

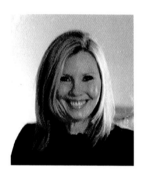

ANNE ROBERTS

Anne Roberts, founding board member of the New York City Marathon Tribute Committee. Anne was born in New York, New York, at 110 Morningside Drive near West 121st Street. She earned a bachelor's degree in English, graduating from Curry College, a liberal arts college in Milton, Massachusetts. Anne had been a volunteer for over five years at the New York Road Runners Club when Fred recognized her talent and appointed her Elite Athlete Director, which she served as for another twelve years, becoming one of Fred Lebow's closest friends. She did the recruiting, scouting, and negotiating to bring world class athletes to the New York City Marathon and other New York Road Runner Club events.

GEORGE S. MITROVICH

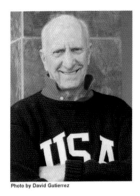

Photo by David Gutierrez

In 2007 he was awarded a Doctor of Human Letters Degree by Point Loma Nazarene University. He served with the Lt. Governor of California as administrative assistant in 1965, press aide to Senator Robert F. Kennedy in the 1968 Presidential campaign, press secretary to United States Senator Charles E. Goodell, Republican of New York, and press secretary to United States Senator Harold E. Hughes, Democrat of Iowa. In addition he worked for two members of the US House of Representatives.

He has written extensively for North American newspapers, including the *New York Times*, *Boston Globe*, *Toronto Globe and Mail*, *Baltimore Sun*, *San Diego Union Tribune*, *Denver Post*, and the *Los Angeles Times*.

His essay on the Boston Red Sox winning the 2004 World Series was featured in the spring 2005 edition of *Elysian Quarterly* (*EFQ*), a baseball literary review.

One of George Mitrovich's speeches, "The Moral Equation," delivered at Boston's famed Fenway Park to a symposium on "The Red Sox, Race, and Jackie Robinson," resulted in a bill to posthumously obtain the Congressional Gold Medal for Mr. Robinson. The bill—the final draft of which was written by George Mitrovich—sponsored by Senator John Kerry and John McCain, passed the Congress and was signed by President George W. Bush. The president presented the medal to Rachel Robinson and her family in a special ceremony at the United States Capitol on March 2, 2005.

It was the teaming with my brother in 1990 to honor Fred by taking him to the Oval Office that helped forge my friendship with him.

This powerful committee of twenty-three helped set the stage for what needed to be accomplished in 1994.

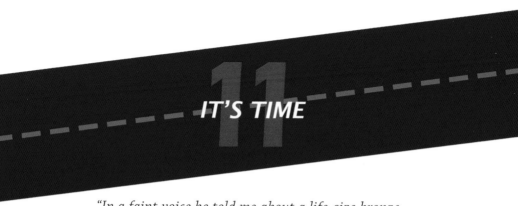

IT'S TIME

IT'S TIME

"In a faint voice he told me about a life-size bronze statue a friend and former runner had commissioned. "It shows me in my running suit and cap, looking down at my watch as if checking a runner's time. The statue's going to be placed at the finish line in time for this year's marathon." Fred said he felt embarrassed. "What have I done to deserve a statue?" "Everything," I answered, taking his hand. "For me and for tens of thousands of others."

—Grete Waitz
Reader's Digest, November 1995

IN FEBRUARY OF 1994 ANNE ROBERTS called to tell me Fred's personal battle was not going so well. He was experiencing recurring dizziness. He felt tired all the time and endured excruciating headaches.

X-Rays confirmed the worst. The cancer had returned, and this time there was nothing to be done about it. Fred's doctors told him straight out that his days were numbered.

Anne was wondering if it was possible to have the statue ready for the upcoming marathon on November 6, which would also be the twenty-fifth anniversary. My response was an immediate yes. Most people would have said no, just can't do it, need money, and November is only eight months away. I just could not give that kind of an answer. It was not in me to tell her no. I knew that Linda and I would find a way to make this happen. But once again here I was, ready to go without funding or approvals in place. No deal with the Parks Department.

Two months later, on Wednesday, April 27, 1994, I flew to New York City and stayed overnight at the Dale Carnegie condo in Jericho, Long Island. The next day I took an early train into Penn Station, took the shuttle over to Grand Central, and changed to an uptown Lexington Avenue train to 86th Street, where I then walked over to the NYRRC at 9 E. 89th Street to see Fred. I loved going into the offices, as there was such a feeling of history. It was here where the real genius took place that created the greatest marathon in the world.

After visiting with Fred, a group of us, which included me, Allan Steinfeld, President and Technical Director of the New York Marathon, and Raleigh Mayer, Director of Media and Public Affairs for the New York Road Runners Club, headed over to the Arsenal, headquarters for the New York Parks and Recreation at 830 Fifth Avenue, to once again meet with Henry Stern and two of his staff.

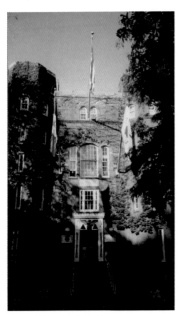

City of New York Parks and Recreation Headquarters

This meeting was to be different than the one I had before. This was a meeting to see if I would get Henry's support for the statue. We were escorted into one of the main board rooms, where Henry held most of his meetings. We were told to take a seat and that Henry would soon be in. A few minutes later he walked in, along with two of his staff.

On one side of the table Raleigh, Allan, and I sat. Allan said to me that I should sit next to Henry, as this was my meeting. Across from us were two of Henry's staff. Henry took the seat to my right at the head of the conference table, his legs crossed. I could see under the table and Henry did not have his shoes on. His big right toe was protruding through his sock. I thought, wow, Henry is really something, an eccentric to the max. His toe may have stuck through his sock, but he was the genius in the room.

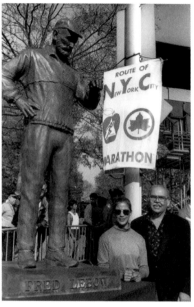

Different than my previous meeting, Henry wanted to know a little bit more about me and said that, since the last meeting I'd had with him, the name Mitrovich came up in his mind a few times. He was not certain why and wanted to know if I had a brother.

Executive Director of Art Commission City of New York, Vivian Millicent Warfield, Sculptor Jesus Dominquez

I shared with him that my brother George had worked for US Senator Bobby Kennedy (NY) in 1968 when he was making his run for the Presidency, and that he also served as press secretary to New York's former United States Senator Charles E. Goodell, who was appointed to replace the Senator after the assassination. (It is the late Senator's son Roger S. Goodell who now serves as Commissioner of the NFL.) This helped start the conversation off in a very good manner. Henry said that two of Senator Goodell's sons actually lived in his building in Manhattan.

Henry then got right to the point. He said, "I endorse the concept of placing a statue of Fred Lebow somewhere here in New York City." He then asked if I would be open to placing the statue in a different location other than Central Park.

I told him I would be open to discussion, but my number one choice would still be in the park.

Henry Stern then suggested we should begin looking for a permanent location somewhere along the 26.2-mile marathon route. He said he would arrange for me to meet the next day with Jonathan Kuhn, the Curator of Monuments for the New York City Parks Department.

We left really happy and excited. We considered Stern's endorsement for the concept to be a major step forward.

The next day at City Hall I met with Vivian Millicent Warfield, Executive Director of the New York City Art Commission.

In my meeting with Ms. Warfield, she told me that one of the first things she had done, upon assuming her position in 1991, was learn about the maquette of Fred Lebow that had been unveiled at the Waldorf Astoria in October of 1991 and my announcement that someday there would be a life-size statue of Fred standing in New York's Central Park. She was very enthusiastic and very encouraging. She laid out some ideas and strategies that I most certainly would need if I were to place the statue in Central Park. We met for almost an hour, and I left her office in a very excellent mood.

I then traveled up to the Arsenal one more time to meet with Jonathan Kuhn. We talked in some detail about finding the best place on the marathon route for placing the statue. I also gave him some

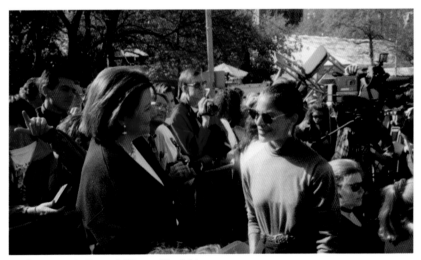

Linda Mitrovich, Vivian Millicent Warfield

information on the members of the Tribute Committee and promised to send some material about our artist, Jesus Dominguez. I was pleased that Kuhn also seemed receptive to our plans for the statue.

Before flying home on Sunday to San Diego, I entered the NYRRC Roosevelt Island May Day 10K. Start time was 10 a.m. Just before we started we had a tremendous thunderstorm and all of us runners had to take shelter. Roosevelt Island is a nice place to run. It is totally flat and surrounded on all sides by water.

After the run I headed back to Jericho and then headed out for a 5:15 p.m. flight from JFK back to San Diego with the knowledge that Henry Stern now accepted the concept of the placement of the statue. I also carried a briefcase of paperwork, including a copy of the "Guidelines for Donating Works of Art to the City of New York." Now that I had Henry Stern's word on the acceptance of finding a place for the statue, the good meetings with Jonathan Kuhn and Vivian Millicent Warfield, and seeing Fred, I was beginning to see that it may be possible to have the statue ready for November.

FRED KEEPS FIGHTING

For a while it seemed that Fred's will and strong work ethic would help him defeat the cancer just as he had done in 1990. He went into the office every day. He kept running. When he became too weak to run, he walked for two or three miles each day.

But despite all Fred's efforts, it soon became clear that the cancer was winning. Weight dropped off his already-thin frame. Dark circles formed around his eyes, and he seemed constantly confused.

Still, he invested every bit of strength into making sure the 1994 Marathon was going to be the best yet. Once Fred ended one marathon, he started planning the next. He always wanted to make the next one better than the one just completed.

On August 8, 1994, Commissioner Henry Stern authorized the issuance of a temporary permit to display the sculpture of Fred Lebow by artist Jesus Ygnacio Dominguez for a period of three days, beginning on

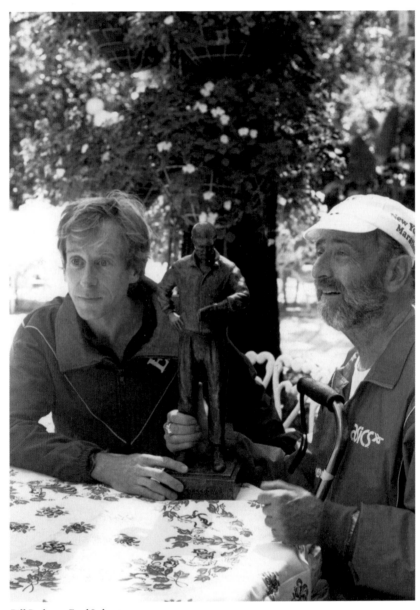

Bill Rodgers, Fred Lebow

Friday, November 4 through Sunday, November 6, 1994, with additional time allotted for installation and disassembly.

I received a signed letter dated August 23, 1994, from Jonathan Kuhn confirming the phone conversation he had with me on August 19 when he told me of the signed agreement by Commissioner Stern.

It was signed by Henry J. Stern, Parks Commissioner, and sent to: Elizabeth Barlow Roger, Central Park Administrator, Parke Spencer, Press Secretary, and Vivian Warfield, Executive Director, Art Commission.

Within a short eight days, we organized a press conference to be held at The Tavern on the Green in Central Park, announcing the upcoming unveiling of the statue.

The press conference had to be done now, as Fred was not doing well. We could not wait any longer, as there was no guarantee that he would be around for the unveiling of the statue.

So on August 27, Linda and I flew to NYC. It was time to hold the press conference with Fred!

On August 30 the New York City Marathon issued a press release stating that a press conference would be held at the Tavern on the Green restaurant to announce that on Friday, at 12 noon, November 4, two days before the twenty-fifth anniversary of the New York City Marathon, a life-size statue would be unveiled at the finish line.

Parks Commissioner Henry Stern, Allan Steinfeld, Bill Rodgers, Linda, and I announced the unveiling to the media.

The happiness on Fred's face showed how excited he was that the statue of him actually was going to happen. Just watching him with Billy Rodgers was absolutely wonderful. Just two friends, together, who gave so much to the sport of the Marathon. The two of them with the maquette of the statue was all the reward we needed for doing all this.

After the press conference Fred, Allan, Bill, Linda, and I grabbed some lunch, and later we all went to dinner.

Fred never knew I was only given a three-day permit to exhibit the statue by the Parks Department. This was the last day Linda and I ever saw Fred; he died on October 9, 1994, forty days after the press conference and twenty-seven days before the unveiling.

STATUE MAKING 101 ADVANCED

"My sculpture is not high art. It is simply a portrait of a man who did so much for so many."

—Professor Jesus Ygnacio Dominguez
Sculptor of the Fred Lebow statue

A FTER DOING THE PRESS CONFERENCE, IT was back to San Diego. This time the pressure was really on, as we had but sixty-seven days to get the statue finished and somehow to New York.

If I thought the last three years were difficult, they were nothing compared to the next sixty-seven days.

VISIT TO STATUE

My first phone call after coming back home was to Jesus Dominguez about how soon the statue would actually be ready so I could arrange to get it to New York. I asked if we could come out to San Diego State University and see the progress. Of course he said yes but for me not to get too discouraged. The statue was in the last steps, which meant it still would be in pieces and not ready to be put together.

Linda and her son Matthew, my daughter Marissa, and I drove out to the school to see the progress. Wow, I had no idea what actually went into this process. Nor was I aware until that day that the mold could break.

We had no time for mistakes!

There were pieces of the statue everywhere and I was very concerned. We took some pictures and Jesus assured me not to worry.

HUGE PROCESS

It was a huge process of putting this statue together from the hollow wax legs from the rubber mold to the hollow wax torso. Bronze ingots being preheated before being put into a crucible and the bronze being poured at 2200° - 2300.° Connecting torso and legs and sandblasting the figure.

The last steps took us into the last three weeks of October, only fourteen days before the statue was to be unveiled in Central Park. We still had much to do from our end! And still no money.

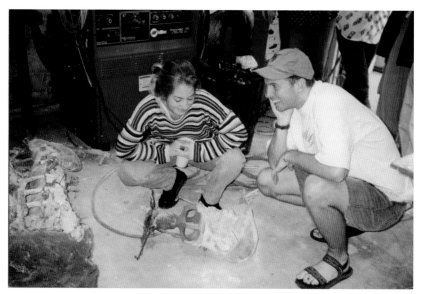

Marissa Mitrovich, Matthew Brannon

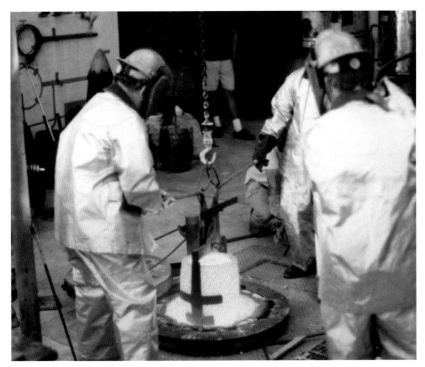

Foundry work

CALIFORNIA TO NEW YORK

I needed to arrange passage for the statue to New York, and for this I phoned Continental Airlines. Continental had served for many years as one of the main sponsors of the Marathon. They were happy to help. I was connected to Continental Cargo, and they offered to donate the transportation of the statue to Newark International Airport.

But first I needed to get the statue from San Diego to Los Angeles International Airport (LAX).

I called my good friend Roger Hedgecock, former mayor of San Diego, who now has one of the most successful radio talk shows in that city. I told Roger what I needed and he invited me to go on his show and tell the community of San Diego that I needed help.

On October 26, two days before the statue was to be flown to Newark, I went on the air and told my story. I gave our office phone number for people to call if they could help. Right after I went off the air, I called our office to hear that, within minutes of me going on the air, our office had received several phone calls from people offering to help get the statue to Los Angeles.

The staff was so excited!

It was just so gratifying to get all those calls. Once again I was filled with gratitude at how willing people are to help each other. We could not have moved the statue one inch without help.

One of those calls was from Electronic Transport Systems, a professional hauling company. I called them immediately and thanked them for offering. I then called Jesus Dominguez and asked exactly what time he expected the statue to be ready. He told me around 5:30 p.m. on Friday, October 28. I then phoned the transportation company and gave them the time and directions to San Diego State and the Art Department where the finishing touches were being done.

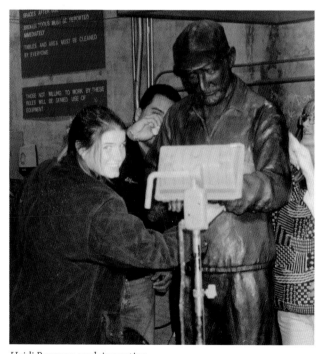

Heidi Brannon applying patina

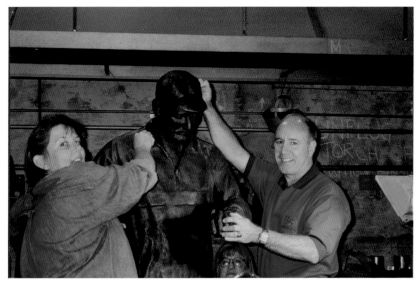

Dan and Linda Mitrovich giving a final shine to the statue

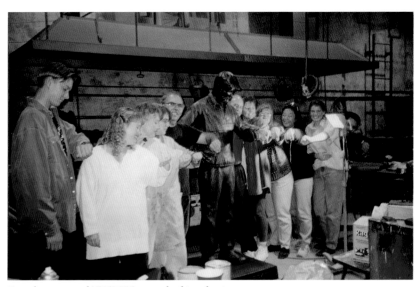

Foundry team and NYCMTC team checking the time

Cargo

Continental Airlines, Inc.
Continental Cargo
Suite 300
15333 John F Kennedy Boulevard
Houston TX 77032

CONTINENTAL CARGO
SPECIAL SERVICES REQUEST

DATE: October 24, 1994

TO: Ken Kramer - LAXFF

CC: Ed O'Meara, Gary Jacobs, Kathleen Yarborough

FROM: Dawn Connor/Manager Cargo Marketing

This is your authorization to ship a bronze statue at no charge from Los Angeles to Newark. The shipper is Dan Mitrovich of the New York City Marathon Tribute Committee. The shipment is approximately 625 lbs. in total weight, and measures 90" x 36" x 36". Mr Mitrovitch or his trucking agent will be tendering the shipment in Los Angeles on Friday, October 28. The statue must be available for pick-up in Newark on October 31.

Please contact me once the shipment is tendered with the air waybill number so that I can monitor the status of this shipment. If you have any questions please contact me at 713/987-6752.

AUTHORIZED BY: Dawn Connor, Manager Cargo Marketing
DATE: October 24, 1994

REGINA

Post-It™ Fax Note 7671

To Dan Mitrovitch	From Dawn Connor
Co./Dept. NYC Marathon	Co. Continental
Phone #	Phone # 713-987-6752
Fax # 619-748-9385	Fax # 713-987-6644

Continental Airlines Cargo Special Services Request

113

House of Representatives
Fred Lebow, Founder of the New York City Marathon

HON. JOSE E. SERRANO
OF NEW YORK
IN THE HOUSE OF REPRESENTATIVES

Friday, June 10th 1994

Mr. SERRANO. Mr. Speaker, I rise to pay tribute to Fred Lebow, the founder of the New York City Marathon, who in this 25th anniversary year of the Marathon, is to be honored with a life-sized statue of his likeness, which will be placed in Central Park this fall.

Mr. Speaker, it may seem only natural, as someone who has lived in New York since childhood and who has had the great pleasure of running in the New York City Marathon, that I would take a special interest in this event. But the New York City Marathon is not simply a source of parochial pride and personal nostalgia. With some 25,000 participants from more than ninety countries around the globe, it is the world's largest marathon, and the model for the dozens of internationally-recognized marathons that have sprung up in the last 20 years.

But Fred Lebow's story is larger than the Marathon. His is the story of an Orthodox youth--born Fischel Leibowitz--who escaped Hitler's meticulous extermination of Eastern Europe's Jews and the Soviet tyranny that followed the War to begin a new life, first in Europe, and then in the United States.

In 1969 Fred Lebow was a successful garment manufacturer and a regular on the jogging track that circles New York's Central Park Reservoir. At the urging of a fellow jogger he entered his first race, which was sponsored by the New York Road Runners Club (NYRRC) and wound around Yankee Stadium. Although he finished next to last, he was captured by the exhileration of the sport and soon became an active member of the NYRRC.

The very next year, at Fred Lebow's suggestion and then under his direction, the Club changed the route of its big race, and the first New York City Marathon was held in Central Park.

Mr. Speaker, that first New York City Marathon had only 126 participants. But each year since 1970, under the guidance of its Director, Fred Lebow, the New York City marathon has grown in size and prominence. As President of the NYRRC Fred expanded the Marathon to encompass all five boroughs of New York City. By 1976, its over 2,000 entrants made the New York City Marathon the world's largest. Moreover, some 500,000 people came out on race day to cheer the runners along the course. In honor of these achievements Mayor Abe Beame proclaimed January 12, 1977, Fred Lebow Day.

After 20 years as President of the New York Road Runners Club, Fred Lebow was recently promoted to the Club's Chairmanship. His leadership has seen the growth of the NYRRC from a small group of avid runners to the largest and most active running organization in the world, with a membership of 28,000 members, a program of more than 100 events annually for athletes of all ages and levels of ability, and a full-time professional staff of 45--supplemented by prominent fitness experts--who hold clinics and classes year-round and provide technical assistance to sporting events around the world. In addition, the NYRRC's Central Park Safety Programs give invaluable support to New York City police and park personnel in promoting the safety of all visitors to Central Park.

Mr. Speaker, I am one of the many thousands of people indebted to Fred Lebow and the NYRRC for their encouragement. Grete Waitz, a nine-time winner of the New York City Marathon who ran--and won--her first New York City Marathon at Fred's urging, is another. I hope my colleagues will join me in honoring Fred Lebow, whose likeness is to be unveiled in Central Park this fall.

UP TO THE LAST MINUTE

On Friday, Linda, her daughter Heidi, and I drove out to San Diego State University (SDSU) around 1 p.m. When we arrived we noticed that there was still much to be done to have the statue ready for shipment to LAX. There was a huge team of people from the Arts Department working on the statue, but they needed even more assistance.

Linda, Heidi, and I helped patina the statue. This took a couple of hours and then it needed to dry before polishing.

By then it was way past 5:30 p.m., and as promised, the Electronic Transport Systems truck and their two-man team was already there.

Other small problems occurred, and now it was close to 9 p.m. The entire team joined together to finish polishing Fred, including the two drivers from the hauling company. Finally, it was time for the statue to be wrapped and crated.

At 11:30 p.m. all of us, exhausted, pushed the statue onto the truck.

Once on board, everyone cheered and applauded! After thanking everyone it was time for Linda, Heidi, and I to follow the truck to LAX, which is 124 miles from the university.

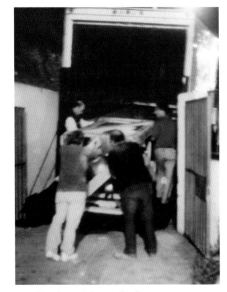

LAX

We arrived at LAX about 1:30 in the morning. Linda and Heidi were sound asleep. I woke them both up so they could watch as we unloaded Fred onto the cargo dock. The shipping crew was ready and waiting for us.

Final loading of the Fred Lebow statue at San Diego State University. Pushing it onto the truck for the ride to LAX and Continental Airlines are Dan Mitrovich, Jerry Dumlau, Jesus Dominquez, and the truck driver.

IN GOOD HANDS

We left the statue in good hands and I started our drive back to San Diego. It was now 2:30 in the morning and I could hardly keep my eyes open. Finally, at about 3:30, I could no longer drive. I was just too tired, so we pulled off the road in Anaheim and checked into the Marriott hotel.

I told the desk clerk to give us a 6:30 a.m. wakeup call, as we needed to get Heidi back for a 9:00 a.m. soccer game. Three hours of sleep is all we got, but we were happy that the statue was on its way to Central Park via Newark International Airport.

Later that day, Saturday, I phoned the Continental Cargo office at Newark to find out if the statue had made it. To my pleasant surprise the cargo person at Newark did not say the statue was there, he said, and I quote, "Fred is here." He went on to tell me that they had been expecting Fred and "Not to worry, Mr. Mitrovich, we are taking great care of Fred." It just brought tears to my eyes when he said it, as it does now as I write it.

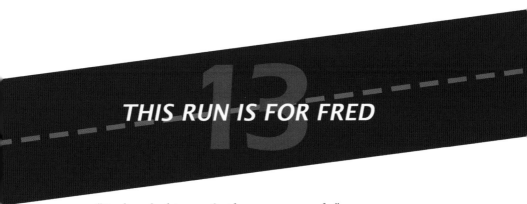

THIS RUN IS FOR FRED

"Fred made this race for the common people."

—Eamonn Coghlan
*Former world record holder in the 2000m and
former world champion in the 5000m*

I FLEW TO NEW YORK ON MONDAY, October 31. Linda and her staff, StephAnnie Hubrecht and Kathy Prince, were to come in on Wednesday. Jesus Dominguez and his wife, Mary Lynn, flew in, too. We were in the city, ready to celebrate the unveiling of the statue—which we delivered as promised to Anne Roberts. It was a major accomplishment for us to deliver the statue, as well as our own accomplishment of doing it in just sixty-seven days.

The company of Racine Berkow and Associates transported the statue from Newark to Manhattan on Tuesday to be placed in storage until Thursday, when it would be brought to Central Park and the Finish Line.

"THIS RUN IS FOR FRED" BOOTH

We were so rushed we had no time for fundraising. We expected corporate sponsors and donors would be excited about the statue and

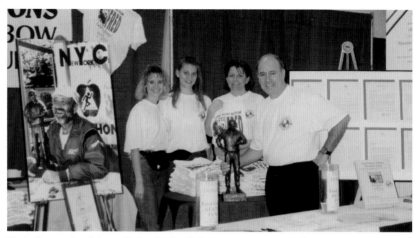

Kathy Prince, StephAnnie Hubrecht, Linda Brannon, Dan Mitrovich

appreciate our efforts enough to want to help us with the debt. Well, we were wrong on that one.

On Thursday we set up our booth at the New York Marathon Expo. We had created T-shirts which said, "This Run is for Fred!" to sell to help raise money. This was no small undertaking by any means.

We had many blown up photos of Fred, as well as the T-shirts and a jar to collect donations for the New York City Marathon Tribute Committee. Our booth was very popular. It became the place for people to share their personal Fred Lebow stories with their families, friends, and us in many languages.

They loved our T-shirts. We sold out. And many were also giving to our donation jar.

All was going fine until one of the Expo people decided that we should not be allowed to get donations at the booth and came and took our donation jar off the table. Without asking, they just took it. Our team was just shocked and sadly disappointed. We could not figure it out. We had come almost three thousand miles on our own expense. We paid for and created our own T-shirts to raise money, paid for everything we were doing, and now the Expo manager from the NYRRC took our donation jar. We were just stunned.

I was filled with anger as I saw the look on the faces of Linda, Kathy, and StephAnnie. How could they, and why did they? I decided not to have a confrontation with the man who took it, as that would be horrible and I did not want to upset our team any more than they already were.

I began to look for Allan Steinfeld, as he could overrule the Expo manager. I found Allan and we set up a meeting with the person who took our jar. The meeting was a short one, as Allan knew he had to reverse the stupidity of what this person had done. It was then arranged for us to keep the jar on the table.

Later in the day on Thursday, we went to Central Park and greeted the arrival of the statue. It was unloaded near the finish line and was tightly wrapped in plastic so you could not tell what it was.

After making certain it was safe, and after talking to the NYPD and Parks Department police about the security of the statue, I felt much better about leaving Fred alone overnight in the park.

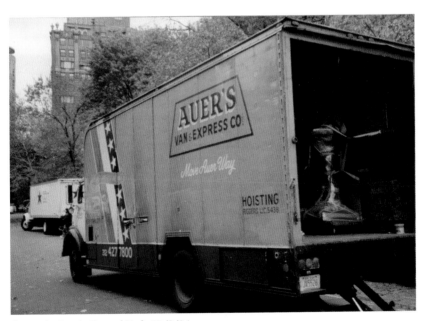

Statue Arrives in Central Park, 11/3/94

PROTEST OF LIFELIKE STATUE

After I got to my room at the hotel, I received a call from Mike Lebov, Fred's brother, whom I had never met. (Mike spelled his last name Lebov and not Lebow.) I was told that the statue could not be unveiled the next day as planned, as the Orthodox rabbi had protested.

In the Orthodox religion there is a ban on the statues of people. It is viewed that statues are a gateway into idolatry, a severe sin in Judaism; however, statues are often viewed differently by other Jewish denominations.

Here we were, twenty-four hours away from the unveiling, and we were told NO! Wow, what else was going to get in our way?

Later Mike Lebov said that if we were to do something to the statue, such as possibly take a small piece out of it, the rabbi would then give his approval. I arranged to meet the rabbi at the statue around 7 a.m. the next morning and bring the sculptor with me. It was just five hours before the unveiling. We removed the plastic and then wrapped Fred in a beautiful blue veil that was handmade by StephAnnie's mother. We made certain that the veil was covering Fred so no one could get a look at the statue until the unveiling. Jesus Dominguez and I went under the veil and Jesus chiseled a little piece out of one of Fred's hands between two of his fingers.

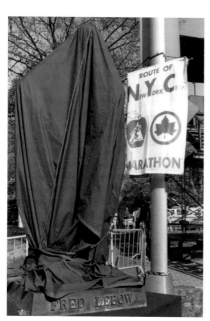

Cover for statue unveiling

The rabbi then inspected and gave his nod of approval. Finally, we were now ready for the unveiling!

You must know that I never met any of Fred's family members until three days before the unveiling. The family did not trust me. All they knew was that I was some runner from California who had a statue made of their brother Fred. This is why I regretted not accepting President George H.W. Bush's invitation for me to step into the photo with Fred and him in the Oval Office on January 31, 1991. Had I done so, the question of who this runner was may have never come up. The fact is, I was an unknown to many in New York.

The day was bigger than we could have ever imagined. Linda and I were so very proud. Exhausted, but so very proud. It was an unseasonably warm fall day—the sky was clear and Central Park was filled with the bright colors of autumn. The statue was covered in blue.

So, finally, three years from the date of the announcement at the Waldorf, we were now only a few minutes away from the big moment. Oh, how we wished that Fred could have been with us. I had to hold back my emotion and not let it get the best of me, as it was time to begin the ceremony.

LARGE CROWD OF FRIENDS, FAMILY, AND RUNNERS

Many of Fred's closest friends and family and admirers were in the crowd: Eamonn Coghlan; George Hirsch; Anne Roberts; John Tope; Tim Murphy; Tracy Sundlum; Muriel Frohman; Paula Fahey Rahill; Photographer Ken Levinson; Jacquelyn Walsh; Raleigh Mayer; Scott Lange; Australian Ambassador to the United Nations Penny Wensley; the Tanzania Ambassador, Mr. Daudi N. Mwakawago; the first woman to run in the Boston Marathon, the legendary Kathrine Switzer; Vivian Millicent Warfield; Allan and Alice Steinfeld and Allan's father, Sam; famed sports artist, LeRoy Neiman; General Manager of New York Athletic Club Leonard Terradista; Jack Rudin; Yokohama International marathoner Keizo Mishima; the President and CEO of Dale Carnegie, J. Oliver Crom; Michael Crom; sculptor Jesus Ygnacio Dominguez and Mary Lynn Dominguez; Tavern on the Green owner Warner L. LeRoy; Managing Director of Tavern on the Green, Thomas W. Monetti; John S. Patterson of Tiffany & Co. ; the President of the Los Angeles Marathon, Dr. William A. Burke; Achilles Track Club founder Dick

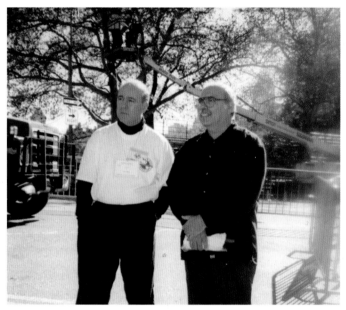

Morning of November 4, 1994, Dan Mitrovich and Jesus Dominquez looking at their accomplishment

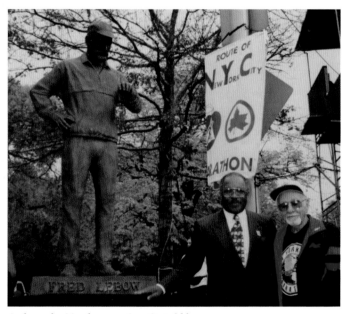

Ambassador Mwakawago, Sam Steinfeld

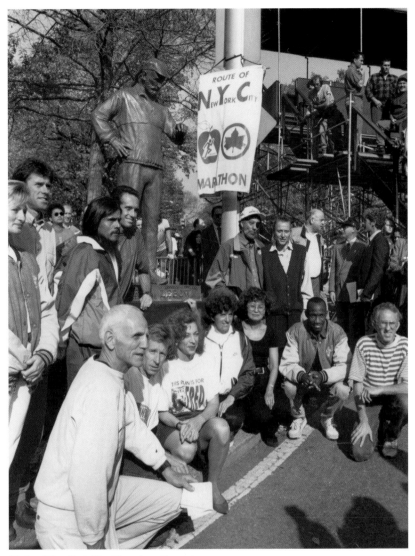

Circle of New York City Marathon Champions:
L-R, Allison Roe, 1981), Rod Dixon (1983), Salvador Garcia (1991), Alberto Salazar
(1980,81,82), Allan Steinfeld, President, Technical Director New York City Marathon,
Grete Waitz (1978,79,80,82,83,84,85,86,88)
Sitting L-R, Norman Higgins (1971), Bill Rodgers (1976,77,78,79), Kathrine Switzer
(1974), Priscilla Welch (1987), Miki Gorman (1976,77), Douglas Wakiihuri (1990),
Sheldon Karlin (1972)

Traum; Marathon runners and past winners of the New York City Marathon, including: Nina Kuscsik (1972–73); Gary Muhrcke (1970); Norman Higgins (1971); Kathrine Switzer (1974); Miki Gorman (1976,77); Rod Dixon (1983); runner-up that year, Geoff Smith; Ingrid Kristiansen (1989); three-time winner Alberto Salazar (1980,81,82); Gianni Poli, who won in 1986; four time NYCM Champion Boston Billy Rodgers (1976,77,78,79); NYCM Champion Grete Waitz, who ran her first NYCM in 1978 and ran for twelve years, winning nine times (1978,79,80,82,83,84,85,86,88); Sheldon Karlin, who won in 1972; Tom Fleming (1973); Norbert Sander (1974); Orlando Pizzolato (1984); Priscilla Welch (1987); Allison Roe (1981); Steve Jones (1988); Douglas Wakiihuri (1990); Wanda Panfil (1990); Liz McColgan (1991); and Willie Mtolo (1992).

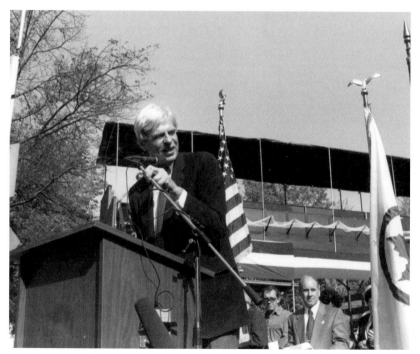

George Plimpton

SPEAKERS AND CELEBRATION

George Plimpton served as master of ceremonies. This was a bittersweet moment for us all, as Fred was not there to see his statue unveiled.

In addition to former winners, there were several hundred runners gathered there to see the unveiling.

Prior to the unveiling, Alberto Salazar, Bill Rodgers, Grete Waitz, Joan Benoit Samuelson, Brian Crawford, Allan Steinfeld, and commissioner Henry Stern addressed the crowd.

Then George introduced me. As I stood behind the podium, Linda went behind the statue to make certain the veil came off without getting stuck. Just as I was ready to start the unveiling, Fred's sister Sara yelled at me, "Dan, you get down here, you did this. I want you to pull the rope to unveil the statue."

Believe me, I wanted to, but I wanted her, her brother Mike, Allan Steinfeld, Brian Crawford, commissioner Henry Stern, and Grete Waitz to do the unveiling.

THE UNVEILING

For a brief moment after the veil was removed from the statue, there was silence. I think people were stunned that the statue looked so much like Fred. It wasn't heroic or larger than life. It was Fred, looking exactly the way so many of us remembered him. The silence quickly gave way to a standing ovation as the crowd poured out their appreciation of their beloved friend.

Many runners touched the statue of Fred for good luck in the marathon to be held the next day. Many left flowers, and many had tears as they missed their friend Fred. Someone stuck a rose in Fred's hand, which has now become a part of the tradition each year at the marathon when Fred is moved to the finish line.

"As much as Fred enjoyed the winners, that wasn't his real passion," said Gloria Averbuch, a longtime Lebow friend who co-authored his biography. "His passion was the thousands [of runners]."

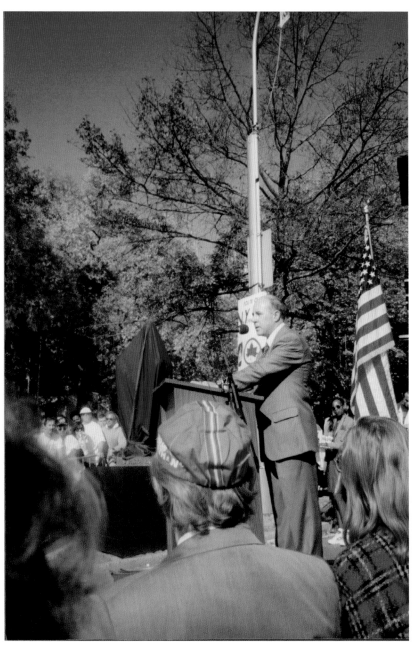

Unveiling Speech, Dan Mitrovich

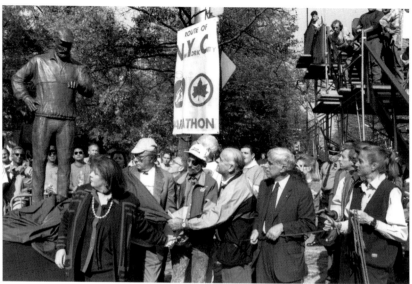

Unveiling L-R:
Sara Katz, Michael Lebov, Allan Steinfeld, Brian Crawford, Henry Stern, Bill Rodgers,
Grete Waitz

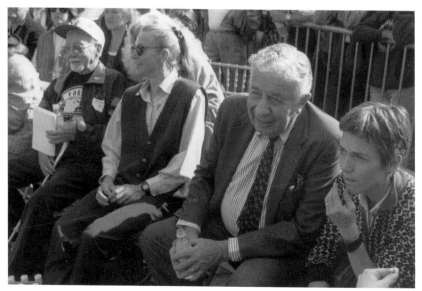

Sam Steinfeld, Grete Waitz, Jack Rudin, Joan Benoit Samuelson

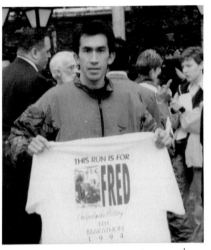

Arturo Barrios, Mexican marathoner, 3rd Place, 1994

"Fred always told the volunteers that every runner was part of the family," said Allan Steinfeld.

Gary Munk of Yonkers said, "You're not peripheral in this race. You're not fringe. You are the core. The fabric of the marathon is (woven) from each individual thread, and every thread is important. That really was how he made you feel. He brought you dignity."

NINETY-SIX HOURS AT THE FINISH LINE

The statue of Fred stayed put for the next ninety-six hours. Fred was there on Sunday, November 6, to welcome champion German Silva of Mexico who won one of the most exciting races in marathon history. Silva defeated his countryman Benjamin Paredes by two seconds. What made his victory even more remarkable was that Silva took a wrong turn about seven-tenths of a mile from the finish line. The champion later told the *New York Times*, "I saw the faces and I knew I had made a mistake. I didn't have to ask anybody." By the time Silva got turned around, Paredes had a forty-yard lead. But Silva caught him within yards of the finish line.

Fred's statue was also there to watch twenty-one-year-old Kenyan Tegla Loroupe win the Women's Division with a time of 2:27:37. Loroupe finished two minutes ahead of the second place finisher, Madina Biktagirova of Belarus, and came within five seconds of tying the course record for a first-time marathoner.

Fred was also there to greet and salute the then-record number of marathon participants—29,768—one of whom was his nephew Moshe Katz, running alongside his coach, Bob Glover.

JOSÉ E. SERRANO
16TH DISTRICT, NEW YORK

WASHINGTON OFFICE:
336 CANNON HOUSE OFFICE BUILDING
WASHINGTON, DC 20515-3216
(202) 225-4361

DISTRICT OFFICE:
890 GRAND CONCOURSE
BRONX, NY 10451-2828
(718) 538-5400

Congress of the United States
House of Representatives
Washington, DC 20515-3216

COMMITTEE
APPROPRIATIONS

SUBCOMMITTEES
LABOR-HEALTH AND
HUMAN SERVICES-EDUCATION
FOREIGN OPERATIONS
EXPORT FINANCING AND
RELATED PROGRAMS

CHAIRMAN, CONGRESSIONAL
HISPANIC CAUCUS

ASSOCIATE MEMBER, CONGRESSIONAL
BLACK CAUCUS

Remarks of the Honorable José E. Serrano
at the
UNVEILING OF THE FRED LEBOW STATUE
in CENTRAL PARK
November 4, 1994

Ladies and gentlemen, so many of the statues adorning our public spaces memorialize historic figures from distant times. Today we gather to unveil a monument to a giant of our own time: Fred Lebow, the founder of the New York City Marathon.

It may seem at times that there has always been a New York City Marathon. Like the Macy's Thanksgiving Day Parade and New Year's Eve in Times Square, the Marathon is a New York City trademark, an annual tradition recognized around the world as the definitive event of its kind.

How strange and wonderful it is then to reflect that this great New York institution grew from its very inception twenty-four years ago to its current prominence under the direction of the man we honor today.

All of us who were Fred's friends and fans are deeply saddened by his untimely passing last month. We miss him, and we miss not being able to share this moment with him. At the same time, however, we know that Fred was aware of these preparations, and that in his modest way he was gratified by this gesture. My deepest thanks go to Dan Mitrovich, the founder of the New York City Marathon Tribute Committee, whose inspiration and tireless efforts made all of this possible for Fred and for us.

Two days from this very moment some of the best distance runners from around the world will be advancing ever closer to this point: the finish line of the New York City Marathon. And as was true for the twenty-four previous runnings of this great race, the form and the spirit of Fred Lebow will be here too.

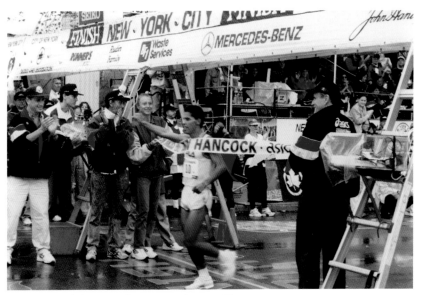
1994 New York City Marathon winner, German Silva

INTO THE WAREHOUSE

It was an incredible, amazing event. But the following day the statue was wrapped in rubber and plastic and taken back to the warehouse in Manhattan. When a reporter from the *New York Post* asked me about this, I told her that it was a very sad moment for me. "I knew we only had a three-day permit to have it in the park," I said, "but I was hoping we could've raised the money to have it here permanently."

And, even if we raised the money, the reality was we had a lot of work to do before we could get the approvals needed to permanently place it in Central Park.

The Parks Commission had to approve the location, the city's Art Commission must approve the statue, and the City had to have a guarantee that there would be money in escrow for maintenance and upkeep.

FOREVER AT THE FINISH LINE

The *Post* also interviewed Fred's brother Mike, who talked about the emotions he felt when he first saw the bronze statue. "I think there are more tears in my body than blood, and I think my brother should stay forever at the finish line," he said.

CALIFORNIA, HERE I COME

Placing Fred in the warehouse bothered me a lot. That statue had been made to be seen, not stand in a dark, musty warehouse collecting dust. In January of 1995, two months after the November 4, 1994, initial unveiling, I decided

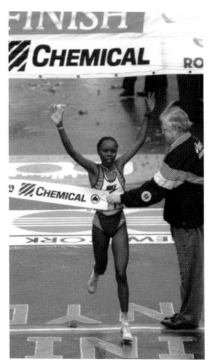

Tegla Loroupe, winner (1994) 2:27:37, (1995) 2:28:06

to call Dr. Bill Burke, co-founder and president of the Los Angeles Marathon.

Bill had known Fred for years. In fact he and Marie Patrick had gone to Fred for advice when they wanted to start a marathon in Los Angeles after the 1984 Olympic Games there.

TENTH ANNIVERSARY, LOS ANGELES MARATHON

"Bill," I told him, "Fred is still locked in the warehouse."

Bill responded, "Why don't you bring him out to Los Angeles for the Marathon and Expo."

I thought that was a great idea. But I had one serious problem. I could not afford to cover the expenses. Bill made a $5,000 donation to the NYCMTC to cover the expenses.

Bill Burke also responded by sending out a press release on January 16, 1995.

> "It is preposterous that the New York Parks Commission would deny a home for the statue of a man who unconditionally gave so much to the city of New York."

Burke credited Fred for a large part of the Los Angeles Marathon's success. "Without Fred Lebow, the City of Los Angeles Marathon would not be what it is today. Fred was a good friend to me, and I am not going to let his memory be locked away in a warehouse."

"FRED LEBOW ON RUN AGAIN"

On March 1 the statue was flown to LA and then exhibited at the LA Marathon Runner's Expo. All went well and, press-wise, maybe better than expected. It seemed that Fred the statue, like Fred in real life, had a penchant for wandering off.

Here's how the *New York Daily News* told the story:

> Fred Lebow is on the run—again. A statue of the late founder of the New York City Marathon disappeared in Los Angeles during a 26-mile race last weekend, leaving red-faced officials pounding the pavement for clues to its whereabouts.
>
> The 550-pound, life-size bronze of Lebow was to make three appearances during the Los Angeles Marathon's 10th anniversary. The movers managed to get the statue to the Marathon Expo Thursday, but its Los Angeles handlers never got the sculpture to scheduled stops at a 20th Century Fox dinner Saturday and at the finish line yesterday.
>
> Local Lebow fans, however, aren't too worried. 'Every marathon, Fred often would just slip off somewhere, either to a private event

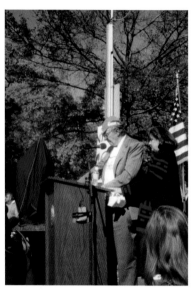

*Fred Lebow's brother Mike Lebov and
sister Sara Katz*

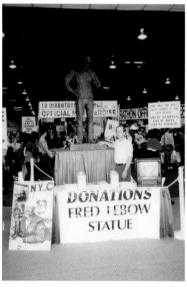

*NYMTC Board of Directors
Dr. Keith Jeffers,
Expo booth, Los Angeles Marathon*

or to go get a slice of pizza,' said Raleigh Mayer, a spokeswoman for the New York Road Runners Club.

'He would just vanish into the sidelines, so this is in keeping with his spirit,' she said. Dan Mitrovich, an ex-New Yorker—who is the person behind the statue, said: 'It's in good hands. Somewhere. We just don't know where. Fred always did things differently. He's got to be up there laughing right now.'

We managed to find Fred a day after the Los Angeles Marathon, locked in a truck near the finish line. We then shipped him back to New York where, sadly, he went back into the warehouse.

14

IN NEED OF AN ANGEL

The man who created Maxwell's Plum, The Russian Tea Room, and Tavern on the Green, Warner L. LeRoy, was our Angel!

—*Daniel S. Mitrovich*

Y OU NEVER KNOW WHO MAY WALK UP TO YOUR TABLE

Looking back on Sunday, November 6, 1994, the day of the New York City Marathon, the Tribute Committee set up a table near Tavern on the Green to sell T-shirts and seek donations to help us honor Fred. Our team of Linda, Kathy, StephAnnie, the CEO of Dale Carnegie, J. Oliver Crom, and I were all there in the rain and the cold late into the day. It was, however, such an exciting time listening to all the Fred Lebow stories. So many runners came to tell us their own personal experience with Fred, and many of the Central Park personnel, including members of the NYPD, came by to share stories about Fred.

Many of the NYPD credited Fred with helping to clean up Central Park. Runners and walkers and the New York Road Runners Club events and activities in the park made the park so much safer. Jackie Kennedy often walked around the 1.58 mile reservoir that was officially named the Jacqueline Kennedy Onassis Reservoir on July 22, 1994.

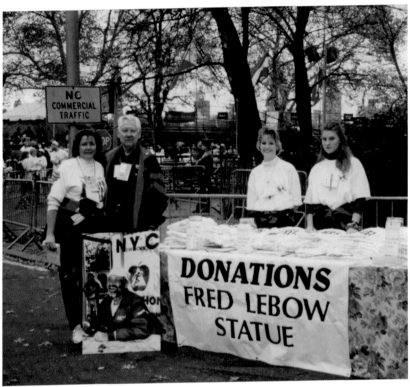

Linda Brannon, J. Oliver Crom, Kathy Prince, StephAnnie Hubrecht

Hearing all those stories told about Fred was so wonderful and made all of us so proud of the work we did to honor him.

As the afternoon grew on, the clouds started to part, and we could see the sun setting over to the west toward California. We knew that in the next two days we would have to go back home. We were leaving Fred in the warehouse, and we did not know for certain how or when we would be able to bring the statue out again.

NEEDED AN ANGEL, WE GOT TWO!

Just before we started to pack it in for the day, two men walked up to the table and introduced themselves to me. One was Warner LeRoy and the other was Thomas W. Monetti. Mr. Monetti was general manager of

Tavern on the Green. Mr. LeRoy was the famous restaurateur and owner of Maxwell's Plum and Tavern on the Green, as well as The Russian Tea Room, three of the more famous restaurants in the world. His daughter Jennifer Oz LeRoy owns Gurney's Montauk Resort & Seawater Spa out on Long Island. Warner was named after his mother's father, Harry Warner, who was one of the founders of Warner Bros. Studios. Warner's father was the famed movie producer-director-actor, Mervyn LeRoy, who was an actor in the 1923 silent film, *The Ten Commandments*. He launched the career of Edward G. Robinson and in 1938 was chosen to head production at MGM. Many considered LeRoy to be one of the greatest directors ever in Hollywood. He was a producer and co-director of *The Wizard of Oz* in 1939 and it was Mervyn LeRoy who introduced Ronald Reagan to Nancy Davis in 1949. Eight of the movies he directed or co-directed were nominated for Best Picture at the Oscars.

There was a star on the Hollywood Walk of Fame, which was located at 1560 Vine Street. (The current site is under construction and all stars have been removed until the project is finished.) Warner LeRoy passed away February 22, 2001, just eight months prior to our final unveiling of Fred.

WARNER LEROY WAS OUR FIRST ANGEL

We talked for several minutes about Fred Lebow and the statue that was now packed away in a storage center. It was Warner LeRoy who came up with an idea to get Fred moved out of the warehouse.

Mr. LeRoy said that a friend of his, a Mr. Ponte, had stopped by earlier and asked him to give me his private phone number. He said Ponte was a well-known businessman who owned quite a bit of property in Manhattan. He suggested that if we needed money for the statue to give Mr. Ponte a call. I called Mr. Ponte early the next week, and to my surprise I actually reached him.

He told me he was there at the Tavern on the Green the day we unveiled the statue of Fred and also on marathon day when we were selling T-shirts. He told me to send him a packet of information on our effort to get the statue of Fred Lebow placed in Central Park.

OUR SECOND ANGEL

I sent it right away via Federal Express.

I then waited a couple of days to phone him so I could ask him what he thought of the material. After that call I telephoned him another forty-four times over the next five months, never being able to reach Mr. Angelo Ponte again until my forty-fifth call when I was finally able to get him on the phone.

When he came on the line, he said, "Daniel Mitrovich, you are one of the most persistent people I have ever met."

He asked me how much money we needed to bring the statue out and back into Central Park. Without hesitation, I said $85,000.

Earlier, thanks to Warner LeRoy, I was able to work out an agreement with New York Parks Director Henry Stern and Executive Director of the Art Commission for the City of New York Vivian Millicent Warfield to place the statue on the Tavern's property which overlooked the finish line of the marathon. I let Mr. Ponte know that on June 27 there was to be a Chemical Bank Corporate Challenge with their spokesperson, Grete Waitz, and 10,000 woman runners finishing up at the Tavern on the Green, and that was when I wanted to rededicate the statue of Fred Lebow. Mr. Ponte told me to call the next day and ask for Charlie Jacobson.

When I did as he instructed, I reached Mr. Jacobson, who was Chief Financial Officer of Ponte & Sons. He had been expecting my call.

When I explained the situation, he said the company had just spent a large amount of money on a dinner to honor Vincent J. Ponte, Angelo's son, who had been named as the recipient of an annual award given by the Italic Studies Institute. Because of that, he said, Ponte & Sons was not able to donate the full amount we needed. Instead, they would donate $50,000 and loan us the other $35,000.

He asked how soon I needed the check and I asked, "Can you send it by Federal Express for next day delivery?"

I'm sure he nearly fell out of his chair. But the rededication of the statue was planned for June 27, and that was only a little over a month away!

I didn't mention it, but there was another reason I wanted the money immediately. The next day, May 18, was Linda's birthday, and I wanted

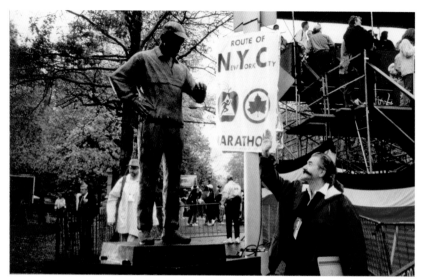

LeRoy Neiman and Fred

to surprise her by showing her the check. Her little company was in debt from carrying costs associated with the statue, and the donation from Ponte & Sons meant that the Tribute Committee could now reimburse her.

When the check arrived the next day, Linda was in a meeting with the San Diego County Water Authority where she served on the board of directors. I phoned the authority and asked the secretary to have Linda call me about an important matter.

When Linda called a few minutes later, I told her she needed to see me. She said she couldn't, as she was driving north from San Diego to San Bernardino, 107 miles, for another meeting. I explained that it was really important and that I'd meet her near a freeway off-ramp that was on her route.

I was waiting when she arrived. When I walked up to her car, she rolled down the window and I handed her the Federal Express envelope.

"Happy Birthday!"

An enormous smile lit her face when she opened that envelope and saw a check for $50,000 made out to the New York City Marathon Tribute Committee.

She just could not believe it. I told her that the committee could now pay her back for the thousands of dollars she had loaned us. Yes, it was a great birthday! But, more importantly, it meant we could now handle the cost of the re-unveiling event next month and that Fred was one step closer to standing tall from sunrise to sunset in the park!

PERSONAL AND UNOFFICIAL

JUSTICES' CHAMBERS
100 CENTRE STREET
NEW YORK, NEW YORK 10013

January 12, 1995

JAMES J. LEFF
JUSTICE

NYC Marathon Tribute Committee
13625 Adrian Street
Poway, California 92064

Attention: Mr. Daniel S. Mitrovich

Dear Mr. Mitrovich:

Over the years I have been solicited to contribute toward the cost of portraits to hang in university libraries, in courthouses, etc. Never once have I been asked to contribute toward the cost of a statue.

I have lived for the past forty years across the street from the 90th Street entrance to Central Park, and I have been a member of the New York Road Runners Club almost since its inception (my membership number is 393). I don't have to tell you how much I owe to Fred for his contribution to running, to Central Park and to the New York City Marathon. My enclosed check is intended to demonstrate that gratitude.

Many years ago I was sufficiently interested in the statuary in Central Park to have written a piece about the statues and who sponsored them - everything from Christopher Columbus, Victor Herbert, Samuel F.B. Morse and Walter Scott, to name a few. Fred Lebow's statue will be the first closely identified with the Park. As to where to put it, I suggest the area just below the steps to the reservoir track at 90th Street.

Very truly yours,

JJL:nc
check enclosed

141

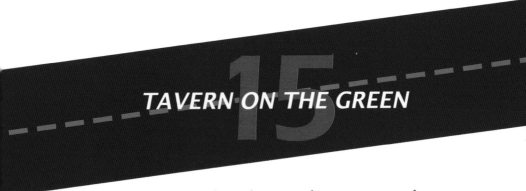

TAVERN ON THE GREEN

"Fred was a good friend to me, and I am not going to let his memory be locked away in a warehouse."

—Dr. William A. Burke
Co-Founder of the Los Angeles Marathon

OUT OF THE WAREHOUSE AND INTO THE PARK

Now that *Angelo Ponte had so* graciously donated the funds, we could plan the event and bring Fred out of the warehouse. As the June 27 event drew near, and with the support of V. Ponte and Sons, I reserved the Crystal Room at Tavern on the Green. I shared with Vincent J. Ponte that we would prepare a blow-up of their check of $50,000 so Angelo could present it to the Tribute Committee during the celebration. I also informed him that Mayor Rudolph Giuliani would be in attendance, as would many other celebrities and well-known runners.

We had much to do for the ceremony and, once again we were planning this 3,000 miles away.

I personally invited LeRoy Neiman and his wife, Janet, and a number of other prominent New Yorkers. Allan Steinfeld and Anne Roberts were most helpful to us and, of course, the staff at Tavern on the Green under the direction of James Stewart, the catering manager for our event, who went above and beyond to assist us in our every need.

Then, on the morning of June 27, the statue of Fred Lebow was brought out of the warehouse and into the park at Tavern on the Green near the finish line of the New York City Marathon.

Linda, our son Luke, and our trusted staff person StephAnnie got to the Tavern early so we could organize for the event. Our evening began with none other than George Plimpton, who had agreed to serve as master of ceremonies.

There were other wonderful people who offered to help whenever I called them. George Hirsch, Bernie Cooper, Scott Lange, Raleigh Mayer, Cara Taback, Muriel Frohman, Harold Stevens, and of course Henry Stern, Commissioner of the New York City Parks and Recreation Department; Jane Rudolph, Director of Public Information; Jack Linn, Assistant Commissioner of Citywide Services; Karen Putman, Central Park Administrator; Toby Bergman, Deputy Administrator Chief of Operations; Karen Lemmey, Monuments Coordinator Art & Antiques; Jocelyn Aframe, Public Information; Sean Williams, Public Information;

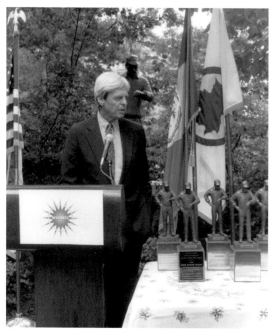

Master of Ceremonies George Plimpton

Craig Konieczko, Public Information, and other Parks and Recreation personnel. Also of course, Vivian Millicent Warfield, Executive Director, Art Commission for the City of New York. These were just a few, but they all played a part in bringing this day to a reality.

I wanted to make sure everything went just right on this special occasion. Although it was not to be the final placement of the statue, it was a huge step toward gaining the support of important people in New York and in the running community. Grete Waitz being on board was huge, as was the support of Mayor Giuliani. It meant that Fred Lebow would be, as printed in the *USA Today Sports Weekly* on May 27 by writer Dick Patrick, "Forever at the finish line."

The evening of June 27, 1995, began with a reception in the Crystal Room at Tavern on the Green.

We then made our way out to the crowd of runners and others who had gathered for the event. George Plimpton, our official master of ceremonies, took his place behind the podium directly in front of the Fred Lebow statue. George began by saying, "I think the only thing wrong with the representation of the statue here is that it is not in motion. Those of you who remember Fred Lebow will remember him as being in motion, not only as a human but in organizing one of the great perpetual motion movements in the history of running, namely the marathon."

I then introduced Allan Steinfeld, president of the New York Road Runners Club, who introduced Grete Waitz, Mike Lebov (Fred's brother), and Sara Katz (Fred's sister). I then introduced Estee Stimler (Fred's niece).

My uncle Fred was the embodiment of the American dream. The proverbial immigrant made good. He took an intangible, unbelievable idea and made it work.

He tried to get people to compete, not with their fellow runners, but with themselves.

—*Estee Stimler*

I had this quote engraved on the plaque placed on the first Fred Lebow

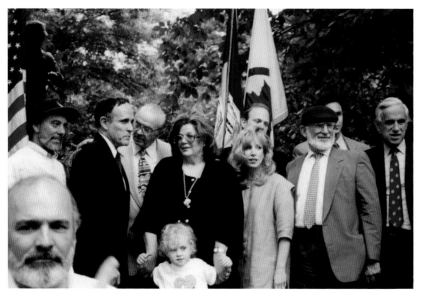

Allan Steinfeld, Mayor Giuliani, Mike Lebov, Sara Katz, Estee Stimler, Manny Katz,
Henry Stern

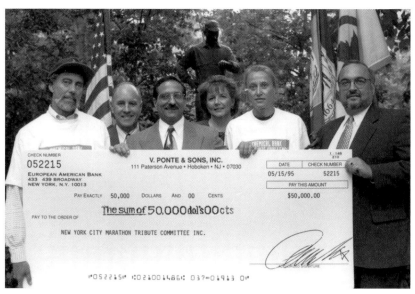

Presentation of $50,000 check. Allan Steinfeld, Dan Mitrovich, Vincent M. Ponte,
Linda Brannon, Grete Waitz, Vincent J. Ponte

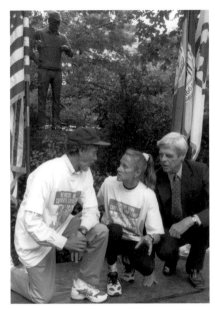

Allan Steinfeld, Grete Waitz,
George Plimpton

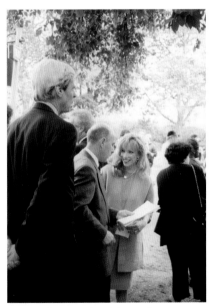

George Plimpton, Dan Mitrovich,
Estee Stimler

replica statue that was to be presented to President Clinton at the White House on October 27, 1995. After the beautiful remarks by Fred's niece, Estee, Vincent J. and Vincent M. Ponte presented an enlargement of the check for the $50,000 donation by V. Ponte & Sons, payable to The New York City Marathon Tribute Committee.

It was then that Allan and I presented to Vincent J. Ponte a replica of the Fred Lebow statue to be given to his father, Angelo Ponte.

The fact that Angelo Ponte listened to me on the phone that day in November, never having met me but believing what Fred Lebow stood for, did what few would do, and that was commitment. Not only commitment, but follow through. That is what made the day and allowed us to bring Fred Lebow out of the warehouse.

We then presented a Fred Lebow statue replica to Fred's close personal friend, Dr. Bill Burke. New York City Parks Commissioner Henry Stern was also presented a replica of Fred, as it was Henry who became such a great supporter of Fred Lebow and the New York City Marathon. It was one of the great parts of my life that I actually could call Henry Stern a friend. He called me "Statue Man." I will never forget Henry, and I only hope the people of New York never forget him as well. Who knows, maybe someday someone will place a statue of Henry Stern in the greatest park in the world.

We then made one more presentation to Mayor Giuliani. When we presented the mayor with his replica, he had a few words to say, and I quote:

"The largest marathon in the world, one of the great sports events in our calendar, one of the great events in New York history. Really something that takes New York and projects it all over the country and all over the world, all of this is due to Fred Lebow. This is a very appropriate monument, and every time this race is run, people are going to know who started it and who inspired it, and they are going to remember. Thank you very much, Fred."

—*Mayor Rudolph Giuliani*

Then I had a very special surprise—for Linda. I invited her up to the podium and gave her flowers. Then, Allan Steinfeld presented her with a replica statue of Fred for her service to the Tribute Committee. The inscription read:

> The New York City Marathon, New York Road Runners Club, and the New York City Marathon Tribute Committee thanks Linda Brannon. A tremendous thank you for the outstanding effort in helping to bring about the success of the New York City Marathon Tribute Committee in their effort to honor the founder of the New York City Marathon, Fred Lebow.

Linda was every bit as shocked and surprised as she was the day I showed her that $50,000 check from V. Ponte & Sons.

I couldn't have pulled it off without the help of one of our most trusted employees, StephAnnie Hubrecht. (StephAnnie's mother, Debra, had made the original cover for the 1994 unveiling of the statue of Fred). With StephAnnie's assistance, I had managed to keep the replica statue hidden for several weeks leading up to this moment. The replica was marked Number Two, so I felt that Linda was in good company, since I had already reserved Number One for a ceremony to be held in October at the White House with President Clinton, and Number Three was reserved for Mayor Giuliani.

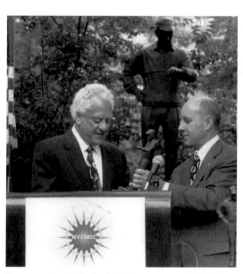

Presentation of Limited edition statue to Dr. William Burke, president of the LA Marathon

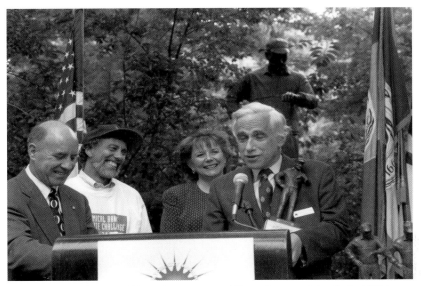

Dan Mitrovich, Allan Steinfeld, Linda Brannon, and Henry Stern receiving Limited Edition statue

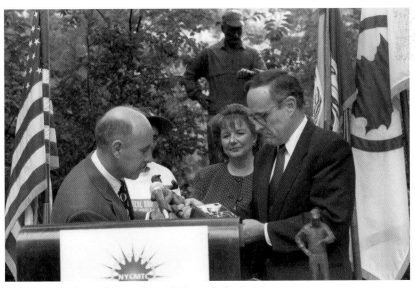

Daniel Mitrovich, Linda Brannon, and Mayor Giuliani

FRED IS BACK

Almost as soon as the statue was rededicated, people started leaving flowers near the statue. Some hung garlands around Fred's neck. Many came by just to touch the statue because they hoped it would bring them good luck. And hundreds of people, New Yorkers and out-of-towners alike, wanted to pose for photographs with the bronze version of Fred.

It seemed to make everyone happy to see Fred at his proper place near the finish line. Friends and acquaintances were thrilled to see him honored. As the years went by, and more people took part in the Marathon who had never met Fred—or who had never even heard of him until they saw his statue—I enjoyed watching them learn about him and come to appreciate him as much as I did.

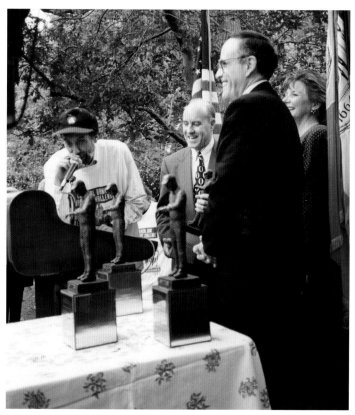

Allan Steinfeld, Dan Mitrovich, Mayor Giuliani, and Linda Brannon

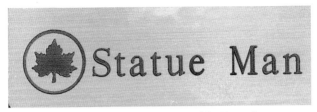

Honor given to Dan Mitrovich (Statue Man) by Henry Stern

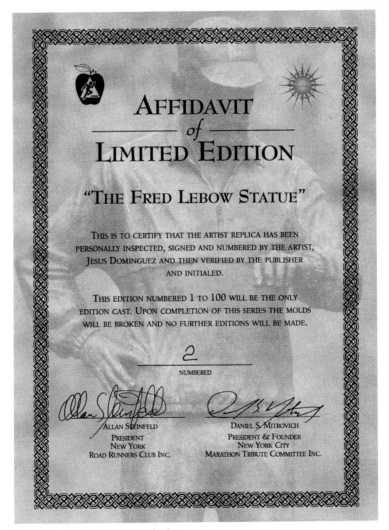

AFFIDAVIT
of
LIMITED EDITION

"THE FRED LEBOW STATUE"

THIS IS TO CERTIFY THAT THE ARTIST REPLICA HAS BEEN
PERSONALLY INSPECTED, SIGNED AND NUMBERED BY THE ARTIST,
JESUS DOMINGUEZ AND THEN VERIFIED BY THE PUBLISHER
AND INITIALED.

THIS EDITION NUMBERED 1 TO 100 WILL BE THE ONLY
EDITION CAST. UPON COMPLETION OF THIS SERIES THE MOLDS
WILL BE BROKEN AND NO FURTHER EDITIONS WILL BE MADE.

2

NUMBERED

ALLAN STEINFELD
PRESIDENT
NEW YORK
ROAD RUNNERS CLUB INC.

DANIEL S. MITROVICH
PRESIDENT & FOUNDER
NEW YORK CITY
MARATHON TRIBUTE COMMITTEE INC.

Fred Lebow Affidavit of Limited Edition

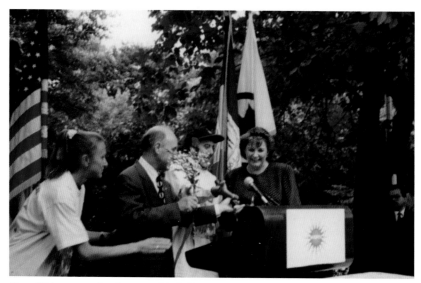

Grete Waitz presenting flowers to Linda Brannon

In November of 1995 Fred was there to celebrate with German Silva and Tegla Loroupe, who repeated their victories of the previous year. This time Silva did not take a wrong turn and shaved twenty-one seconds off his 1994 finish, completing the race in exactly 2:11. Loroupe came across the line seventeen minutes later, at 2:28:06. The following year Giacomo Leone of Italy finished first in 2:09:54, and in 1997 John Kagwe of Kenya captured the first of his two consecutive victories—and the first of three in a row for Kenyan runners—turning in a then-course record of 2:08:12.

Every year Fred was there to celebrate with the winners—and everyone else who managed to keep moving forward for 26.2 miles. And every year I thought, this is the year Fred finally becomes a permanent resident of the park. But it didn't happen.

16 RUNNING WITH THE PRESIDENT

"I choose to keep going, hoping my pounding away, regardless of the news or the weather, would provide some small measure of inspiration to joggers around the country who put one foot in front of the other."

—Bill Clinton

WHILE I PERSEVERED TO FIND A permanent spot for the statue, I continued to enjoy the thrill of long-distance running. Between 1994 and 1997 I ran in the Boston Marathon four more times, finishing with my best Boston time of 3:53:51 in 1995.

One of the most exciting moments for me came, not in a marathon, 10K, or other running event, but at the White House.

It was May of 1995, and as a surprise for Linda, who was to become my wife, I had begun arranging a private run with President William Jefferson Clinton. (Sorry Fred, this one was for me).

I phoned a friend, John B. Emerson, who served as Deputy Director of Intergovernmental Affairs, to help with the process. (John later served as Ambassador of the United States to Germany.) If you think getting a statue placed in New York Central Park was difficult, try arranging to do a private jog with the President of the United States sometime.

But I needed something special to impress Linda, or at least I thought I did. Now, I am sure she would tell you that it was not necessary and that she was in love with me already on account of my good looks, charm, and, of course, wit! Most women know that we men can often produce miracles for the women we love and want to marry, and I was no exception to this statement. (Sorry, men, if I have set the bar a little high for you. But if you need any help, just give me a call!)

Talking to John was the first step of many. I cannot count the number of phone calls, faxes, and people I talked to in order to accomplish this incredible idea of mine for the woman I was in love with and still am to this day!

So, on May 26, 1995, I invited Linda to dinner and told her to bring her own credit cards.

We went first to the Sportmart, a sporting goods store in Carmel Mountain just outside San Diego. I told her what she should buy and not to ask any questions. My plan was to tell her to buy running gear and running shoes, of course. Then, after shopping I would take her to dinner.

Which is exactly what I did. I must tell you she was not happy, as she did not like me telling her what to buy with her own credit card. I took her to a nearby restaurant, and now it was time for the big announcement. Looking straight into her eyes, I said, "Linda Brannon, William Jefferson Clinton, the forty-second President of the United States, has invited you to attend the White House for a special presentation, to be followed by a private jog with him."

She absolutely did not believe me. I told her it was the truth, the gospel truth. Wow, she was just shocked. We started training the next day, May 27.

I had designed a training program for her to take her from running zero miles to being able to run three miles at an eight-minute pace within a five-month training period.

This was very difficult, as she was so busy with work and had not run since college. She trained for a period of four months until we flew to D.C. to jog with President Clinton on October 27, 1995.

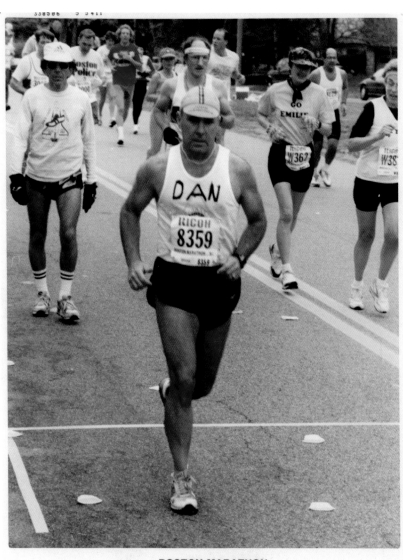

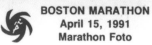
Dan Mitrovich, 1991 Boston Marathon

Arranging for the run was a huge undertaking. I started with John Emerson, and he introduced me to William (Billy) Webster, who served as Deputy Assistant to the President and Director of Scheduling and Advance.

Through the hard work that John, Billy, Margo Spiritus, Stephanie Streett, Anne Wally, Nancy Hernreich, Rebbeca Cameron, Betty Currie, Stephen Goodin, and many others, we made it happen.

However, there had to be an official reason for all this, and I had the perfect one: present the first replica of the Fred Lebow statue to the President of the United States. I also invited Allan Steinfeld, who had succeeded Fred Lebow as president of the New York Road Runners Club, and George Hirsch, publisher of the magazine *Runners World*. The run was scheduled for the morning of October 27, 1995.

The day before the run was scheduled, I took Linda to 221 Russell Senate Office Building, Office of US Senator Joseph R. Biden Jr., Delaware. Senator Biden and his family are some of my favorite people. Upon entering the senator's office, I asked for executive assistant Marianne Baker, who was expecting us. She took us into the senator's office. It was so great to see Senator Biden.

The friendship began in 1972 when my brother George was serving as press secretary for US Senator Charles Goodell from New York, and Joe was a member of the New Castle County Council. The Council Member was running for the US Senate and came to my brother to ask his support. Brother George was not so certain that the young, twenty-nine-year-old Joe Biden could defeat Senator Cale Boggs, who was a former congressman, governor, and now running for his third term in the US Senate and known to be a Delaware institution. Of course my brother was not alone in that feeling.

My brother told Biden he would have a tough time getting elected. I have come to believe one should never underestimate a Biden. His sister, Valerie Biden Owens, was Joe's campaign manager, brother Jimmy was his finance chair, and brother Frank headed up the volunteers.

The rest is history. At age twenty-nine Joe Biden was elected to the US Senate. One thing that is so great about Senator Biden is his ability to focus on those in the moment and make you feel like a million dollars and then some. He truly makes the moment about you!

We were just getting settled when Joe's secretary, Marianne, appeared at the door and said, "The president's office is on the line."

Biden reached for the phone, but Marianne stopped him. "It's for Mr. Mitrovich," she said.

A surprised smile formed on Joe's face and he gestured for me to take the call.

The woman on the other end of the line introduced herself as Mary Morrison, assistant to Nancy Hernreich, President Clinton's director of Oval Office operations. "Mr. Mitrovich, the president wants to know if it would be all right with you if he invited a close friend of his to run with you tomorrow morning." She explained that Gary Smith, a friend from Arkansas, was in town, and the president would like to ask him to join us. But the president knew this was a special day for me and wanted to be sure it was okay with me before he did. It was really hard to believe

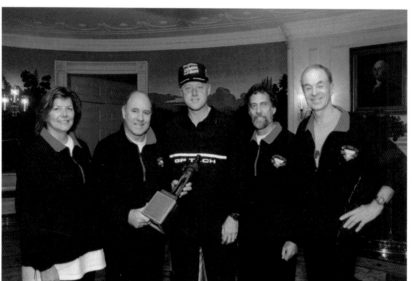

Presentation of Number One limited edition statue to President William Jefferson Clinton in a ceremony at the White House October 27, 1995. Linda Brannon, Dan Mitrovich, President Clinton, Allan Steinfeld, and George A. Hirsch, Publisher, Runner's World

Courtesy of White House Photo Office

that the President of the United States was asking me if I had a problem with him inviting a personal friend of his to join us.

Those who have ever had the opportunity to meet President Clinton know exactly what I am saying. He is just special.

I replied to Mary Morrison, "Of course. That's absolutely fine with me."

Senator Biden jokingly wondered out loud how I had become so important that the president had to seek my opinion before he made personal decisions. Joe certainly had fun with the call.

We visited with Senator Biden for about twenty minutes and he was just terrific to Linda. He was so nice to say such wonderful things about the Mitrovich family to Linda, and he made me feel so very important in the process. My nephew Tim Mitrovich had interned with Senator Biden back in 1984, and my own daughter Marissa chaired the Young Professionals for Senator Biden's Unite Our States in 2005.

Note from Allan Steinfeld to Dan Mitrovich about New York Times photo, November 2, 1995

The next morning at 6:15 a.m. I drove a Hertz rental car to the entrance of the SW Gate of the White House, where our car was searched. We were then permitted to drive up to the rear entrance of the White House, directly outside the International Room. We sat in the car for a few minutes and then someone approached the car, knocked on my window, and invited us in to the Diplomatic Reception Room. Allan, George, Linda, and I walked into the room, and there we were greeted by Major Darren W. McDew, Air Force Aide to the President. Major McDew introduced us to Gary Smith, the personal friend of the president.

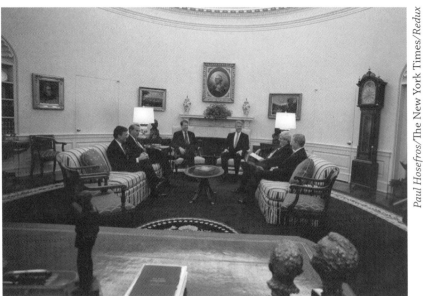

The Fred Lebow statue can be seen on the President's desk in the lower left-hand corner, November 2, 1995.

Also in the room was White House photographer Sharon Farmer.

Exactly fifteen minutes later—right on time—President Clinton walked down from his family's private residence upstairs. The president came over to each of us and welcomed us to the White House. The president was open and very friendly and made us all feel so welcome. We had designed special warm-up jackets and pants for all of us to wear that day. And we presented a set to President Clinton. Much to our delight, and in another act of graciousness, the president changed from his sweats into ours.

Then, in my capacity as founder and president of the New York City Marathon Tribute Committee, I presented the president with the first replica of the Fred Lebow statue.

Clinton was gracious, affable, and remarked about how honored he was to receive the very first replica of the statue. He told his aide to take it up to the Oval Office.

The fact is that a photo appeared in the *New York Times* a few days later, November 2, 1995, and there, right in the middle of a meeting with

President Clinton, Vice President Al Gore, Speaker of the House Newt Gingrich, Minority Leader of the US Senate Tom Daschle, Senate Majority Leader Bob Dole, and Representative Richard A. Gephardt, the congressional minority leader, was the replica statue of Fred Lebow, standing right on a credenza in the Oval Office for all to see. (Thank you, Mr. President, for keeping your word to display it.) After the aide left to take Fred up to the Oval Office, the president said, "Are you all ready to go for a jog?"

Before we could answer, one of the Secret Service agents asked, "Should I have the van brought around, Mr. President?"

Clinton shook his head. "Get the limo and we'll all ride over to Hains Point together."

With an apologetic look on his face, the president explained, "Hains Point is one of the few places they'll let me run these days."

He told us that the Secret Service had tightened up on him since someone had been arrested a few weeks earlier for firing several bullets in the general direction of the White House. Thankfully, no one was hit.

Hains Point was only a short drive from the White House—about fifteen minutes—and we certainly didn't mind taking a ride in the presidential limousine. I found it rather amusing that we were heading to a "remote" area of the city to jog, because we certainly weren't being inconspicuous. There is nothing more exciting than being in a Presidential motorcade, especially when you are with the President of the United States. Our "motorcade" consisted of two motorcycle policemen in front of us, two motorcycle policemen in back of us, and a number of other vehicles, both in front and to our rear. We made so much noise, and caused such a stir, that it would have been pretty easy for just about anyone in the city to know where the president was that morning. The fact is, the citizens of the District of Columbia almost always know when the president is driving by.

Furthermore, we were hardly going to look like your average group of joggers. Especially with those Secret Service agents running alongside us and that helicopter hovering overhead. Several other agents were stationed at various points along our route—in cars, on bikes, and even in a boat on the Potomac River.

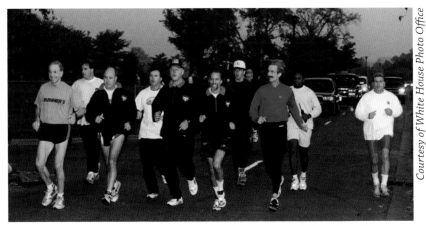

Haines Point run, October 27, 1995. George Hirsch, Dan Mitrovich, President Clinton, Allan Steinfeld, Gary Smith, and Secret Service escort.

I have had the opportunity to meet other former presidents of this country, as well as presidents of other countries, and each time I know just how special that moment is.

When we reached Hains Point, Buckeye Drive, and Ohio Drive SW, we all got out of the limo and began some stretching exercises. Once out of the limousine, we were given instructions in what to do if the president came under attack. We were told to hit the ground and to not look up. We were also told that if any of us could not keep up with the president, we would be escorted back to White House Guest One, which was a white van.

It was a beautiful morning. Calm and clear, but chilly, as an October morning should be. The sun was just beginning its ascent over the city, bringing with it the promise of a short-sleeve afternoon. October is always a beautiful month in the District, eclipsed only by the explosion of color that overtakes the city every spring when cherry blossoms seem to wrap the Tidal Basin in a cloud of pink.

There are no cherry blossoms in October, but the reds, golds, and yellows of fall were everywhere in Hains Point and the surrounding Potomac Park. I had jogged through this park many times during my years in Washington, enjoying its terrific views of the city, and

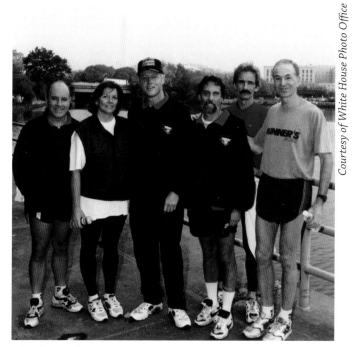

*After the run along the river, Dan Mitrovich, Linda Brannon,
President Clinton, Allan Steinfeld, Gary Smith, George Hirsch*

watching the families who had come to picnic, fish, or ride bikes along the Potomac River.

About halfway into our run, the president turned to me and asked if I had ever seen a statue called *The Awakening.*

I admitted that I hadn't.

"It's one of my favorites," he said. "Would you like to see it?"

Of course I said yes.

He assured us that it wasn't far off our route, but I don't think that would have mattered to any of us anyway. We were all having a fine time being with the president.

The sculpture, which was completed by J. Seward Johnson in 1980, turned out to be one of the most unusual pieces of art I've ever encountered. The piece is about seventy feet long and depicts a bearded giant who seems to be bursting out of the ground. Only his head and portions of his arms and feet are visible, giving the impression that the rest of the body is still buried. It's an amazing piece of art, and the president, in particular, seemed to be drawn to it. It's remarkable and well worth seeing—but you'll no longer find it bursting from the earth at Hains Point. The whole thing was moved to Prince George's County, Maryland, in 2008.

Our jog with the president lasted exactly 28:03 minutes; being the most exciting jog of my life, I wanted to make certain the time was correct. We ran along at a pretty good clip. As I said previously, the president seemed to be in good shape. Although Linda had trained long and hard for this, she simply couldn't keep the pace. She eventually had to take a seat in the White House Guest One van. As we approached the finish, the Secret Service slowed the van enough so she could get out. Linda was able to run and catch up with us, and we finished together.

At one point along Ohio Drive SW, we passed an area where members of the press corps had gathered to take photos and video of the president jogging. A few days later a friend of Linda's told us that he was in an airport, waiting for his flight to Hawaii and idly watching CNN. A story came on talking about the different ways people could get access to the president. Suddenly, there I was, jogging along next to Clinton.

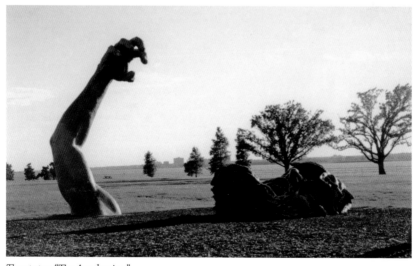

The statue "The Awakening"

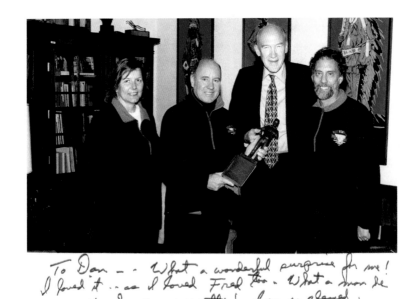

To Dan — — What a wonderful surprise for me! I loved it … as I loved Fred too. What a man he was. You honor me greatly! I am so pleased.

Linda Brannon, Dan Mitrovich, Senator Simpson, Allan Steinfeld

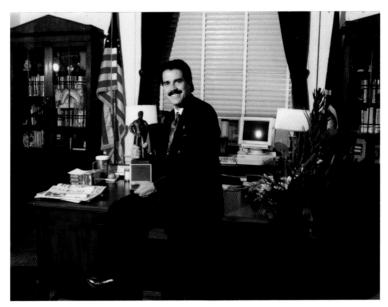

Congressman Jose Serrano

After we finished our jog that morning, the president spent about thirty minutes just visiting with us under the Frances Case Memorial Bridge. As we stood along the river, we talked mostly about running and life in general. The president's runner's watch was broken, so Gary Smith took his off and gave it to the president. We did not engage in any discussion about politics. This was the president's personal time and we respected and appreciated his time that he was giving to us.

We boarded the limousine and started heading back to the White House. On the way back I brought up the subject of an article that had appeared on the front page of *USA Today* that morning. The article had to do with the federal budget and included several graphs prepared by the Office of Management and Budget, the White House office charged with submitting the president's annual proposed budget to Congress.

I thought one of the graphs was confusing and shared my thoughts with the president.

"It needs to be simpler," I said. "Ninety-nine percent of the general public won't be able to understand it."

"How would you fix it?" he asked.

So Linda and I shared with him what we would change.

The president was very engaged in our thoughts. It is not often that one gets to share one's thoughts with the president of the United States in a private setting in the presidential limousine.

STANDING TALL AFTER 9/11

"The attacks of September 11th were intended to break our spirit. Instead we have emerged stronger and more unified. We feel renewed devotion to the principles of political, economic and religious freedom, the rule of law and respect for human life. We are more determined than ever to live our lives in freedom."

—Rudolph W. Giuliani

SOMEHOW, AFTER THE 2000 MARATHON I really knew things were going to change. But I didn't know we were on the verge of a terrorist attack that would shake the American people to the depths of our souls.

Just about everybody remembers where they were on the morning of September 11, 2001. If you're old enough, you'll always recall hearing that terrorists had flown fully-loaded airliners into the World Trade Center and the Pentagon and that another had crashed into a field in Pennsylvania.

The few days prior to the horrendous attacks, Linda and I and our two daughters, Heidi and Marissa, had been enjoying a week-long Caribbean cruise. As far as we were concerned, all was well with the world. We had no inkling that disaster was on the horizon.

If you've ever been on a cruise, you know that often you sit with the same people at your table every night for dinner. We were fortunate to find ourselves at the table with a likeable couple from Texas, Craig and Tammie Cunningham. Craig was a captain with American Airlines.

Over the course of a week, we became pretty close. We exchanged addresses and phone numbers and promised to try to stay in touch. Our cruise docked in Miami on Monday, September 10, and we caught a five-hour flight back to San Diego. By the time we finally got home, we were too exhausted to even unpack, and we headed off to bed.

Early the next morning we were awakened by a phone call from our son Jesse, who asked if the United States had gone to war. I was startled by his question and quickly snapped on the television to see what he was talking about. Linda and I were horrified as we listened to the news reports that American Airlines Flight 11 and United Airlines Flight 175 had crashed into the Twin Towers of the World Trade Center. That mind-numbing information was followed quickly by reports of two other crashes. Terrorists had taken control of American Airlines Flight 77 and flown it into the Pentagon. And United Airlines Flight 93 had smashed into a field near Shanksville, Pennsylvania.

It was only later that the world learned of Flight 93's intended destination—the United States Capitol Building. That plan was thwarted when a number of heroic passengers rose up and attempted to retake control of the aircraft. Of course everyone on board was killed, as was the case in all the other crashes as well.

We felt helpless as we watched the chilling news reports on television and saw the thick, black smoke billowing out of the collapsing Twin Towers. We wanted to reach out, to help someone, to stop the horror— but what could we do?

We watched in a stunned silence for a few minutes. Then I turned to Linda and said, "Maybe we should call Craig."

"Absolutely," she agreed. Neither one of us felt that Craig was one of the pilots, but we wanted to make certain. I grabbed the phone and punched his number.

It rang once. Twice. Three times. I felt my heart pounding in my chest. Then I heard his voice come on the line.

"Hello?"

"Craig?"

"Yes."

"It's Dan and Linda Mitrovich. So glad to hear your voice. When we saw the news, we thought of you and Tammie right away."

"I'm watching it on TV. It's unbelievable."

He thanked us for calling to check on him, and we talked for a few minutes. He told me that he didn't yet know if he had lost any close friends in the attacks, explaining that American Airlines had more than 10,000 pilots. He had been on the phone most of the morning, trying to get any news he could, but information was slow in coming.

I wished him well and told him to keep in touch if there was anything we could do.

A few days after the call with Craig, I received a call from Cristyne Nicholas, chief of staff to Mayor Rudy Giuliani. Cristyne said that Mayor Giuliani wanted to make the statue permanent in Central Park. She said the mayor said it was the right time to do this.

Fred had been standing at the site of The Tavern on the Green, adjacent to the finish line, since June 27, 1995, and now the time had come. It had been ten years since I first announced from the podium at the Waldorf Astoria on that October 31, 1991, date that there would be a life-size statue of Fred standing in the greatest park in the world, none other than New York's Central Park.

We were so moved that Mayor Giuliani was thinking of Fred at a time like this, with everything on his mind and his city just going through the 9/11 devastation.

We also thought that there was not a better time to add Fred to the other monuments in Central Park, as he stood for so much good and made the difference in so many lives. This was exciting news as, finally, we could put Fred into a final place in Central Park.

I immediately called Allan Steinfeld to give him the news and ask him to help select a date for the ceremony. We both felt that the best time to do this would be Saturday, November 3, the day before the thirty-second running of the New York City Marathon.

I let him know that I would confirm with the mayor's chief of staff as soon as I hung up the phone. Since this was a New York City Marathon Tribute Committee program, Linda and I would take care of all the details, as we always had over the past ten years.

Allan asked what he could do, and I reminded him of what I once told Fred Lebow as we both left the White House's Oval Office on January 31, 1991. Fred asked that same question, and I said, "Just show up." I now told Allan to just show up and bring as many runners as he could. I also let Allan know that I still needed more money for the endowment and that I would be shaking all the trees to find it between now and November 3.

About ten days later I received a call from Todd Wissing, a captain for American Airlines and a communications manager. Right in the middle of planning for our big event to be held on November 3.

He told me he got a call from a friend of his who's also a captain with United Airlines. "His name is Mike Burr. Mike came up with the idea of running a flag across America to honor the flight crews of 9/11. He would like to talk to you about helping in Los Angeles. I gave him your number, so would you please talk to him?"

Although we had a huge assignment on our plate, I assured him that I'd be expecting the phone call and that both Linda and I would be happy to do whatever we could to help. Linda and I were honored to think we could play a small part in honoring those who had died and, at the same time, help bring a small measure of healing to a country that was shattered by grief.

Mike Burr called a few days later. He was filled with huge energy and passion to honor the flight crews of both United and American. He told me he was organizing, along with three others, to run an American flag across America, beginning on October 11 at the state capitol in Boston, and ending on November 11, 2001, at Dockweiler State Beach, which is located at the end of the runways of the Los Angeles International Airport. He said he needed help in Los Angeles with VIPs and the staging of the event. I told him we would be honored to help in assisting to make that happen and not to worry, we would take care of it for him and his team.

What Mike Burr was doing was a huge undertaking, as it totaled 3,872 miles from Boston to Los Angeles, and the trip covered nineteen states, including the District of Columbia. He also asked me if I would mind talking to a man named Tom Heidenberger who was a captain with US Airways.

The next day I found a heartbreaking message from Captain Heidenberger on my office voice mail. Speaking in a voice choked with emotion, he told me that his wife, Michelle, had been a member of the crew on American Airlines Flight 77, the plane that had crashed into the Pentagon. He went on to say that he considered her to be a hero and that, in fact, all of the members of all the flight crews were heroes, and they deserved to be honored just as much as the policemen and firemen who had rushed to the World Trade Center in an effort to help victims of the attack.

I called him back right away and told him I'd do everything within my power to see that something was done to properly honor his wife and the other flight crew members who lost their lives on 9/11.

During our phone conversation, my mind started working on how to do something that would honor these heroes.

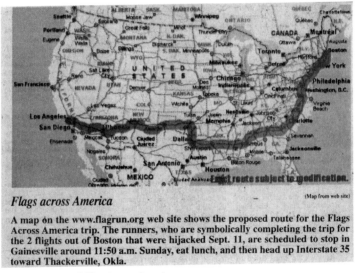

Flags across America   (Map from web site)

A map on the www.flagrun.org web site shows the proposed route for the Flags Across America trip. The runners, who are symbolically completing the trip for the 2 flights out of Boston that were hijacked Sept. 11, are scheduled to stop in Gainesville around 11:50 a.m. Sunday, eat lunch, and then head up Interstate 35 toward Thackerville, Okla.

Americans United Flag Across America

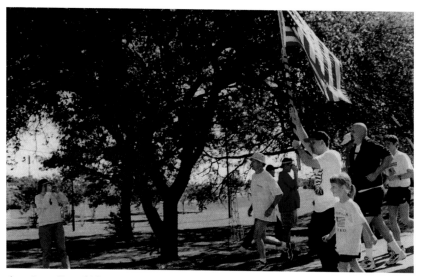

Americans United Flag Across America. American Airlines Captain Craig Cunningham and his daughter Kelsey, Gainesville Daily Register Gainesville, Texas, Jerry Prickett (Photographer), October 26, 2001. The flag still needed to be carried another 1,377 miles to Los Angeles.

After the phone call with Tom, I called my friend Bobby Barrett, who was then General Vice-Chairman of the Tribal Council for the Viejas band of Kumeyaay Indians, and told him, "Bobby, we're going to make the Fred Lebow statue permanent in Central Park." I said that Mayor Giuliani's office called and we had picked November 3, 2001, to be the date for the permanent placement ceremony of the Fred Lebow statue.

I told Bobby that we also needed some additional help with the endowment for the park, one of the conditions placed on our committee to permanently place the statue in the park.

I explained to Bobby that we had paid other sums, but we still needed more money, and the Parks Department needed a check for $25,000 for the endowment. The check should be made payable to the New York City Department of Parks and Recreation.

I also said, "I have an idea. I believe we should honor the flight crews of American and United Airlines who were lost on 9/11, and I want you to be part of it."

I explained that I thought it would be a good idea to combine the ceremony for the statue in Central Park with a tribute to the flight crews of 9/11. I also hoped to involve some members of the Viejas tribe in the proceedings and, perhaps, if I could arrange it, in another ceremony at Ground Zero.

I told him of my phone call with Tom Heidenberger.

Bobby was obviously moved by what he heard. He was a big man with a huge heart. "I like the idea, Dan. Let me talk to the Tribal Council, and I'll get back to you."

As was always the case, Bobby did exactly as he promised. Within a couple of days, he took my request before the Tribal Council, and they gave him the go-ahead. He reported to me that the council felt honored that they could play a small part in finalizing the statue of Fred and, at the same time, honor the flight crew members who had lost their lives.

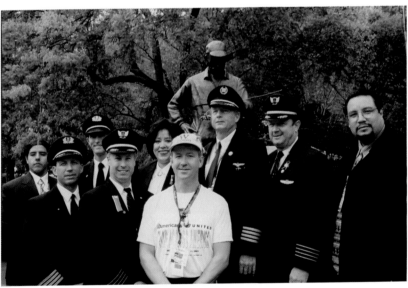

Ral Christman, (Viejas), United and American Airline Crews,
US Airways Captain Tom Heidenberger, Mike Burr, Founder of Americans United Flag
across America, and Bobby L. Barrett, Vice Chairman, Viejas Band of Kumeyaay Indians

Bobby said he would like to come to New York along with Ral Christman, a member of the tribe who was a Bird Singer. Ral planned to perform beautiful songs telling the story of those who have traveled beyond the earth to a new land.

The phone call between Bobby and Linda and I was so very, very special. After the call Linda and I both cried for a few minutes as we thought about how blessed we were to have a friend like Bobby. We were also deeply touched that a Native American tribe wanted to not only honor Fred but do what they could to honor fellow Americans who had died 3,000 miles away.

After finishing my conversation with Bobby, I called both Mike Burr and Todd Wissing and let them know of my phone conversation with Bobbie Barrett, that his tribe had agreed to write a check to the Parks Department of New York City, and that Bobby and the Tribal Council thought it would be a great idea to honor the flight crews at the same time as our final dedication of the Fred Lebow statue.

I also said we would honor Michele Heidenberger at the same time.

They were so excited and moved about the idea. I told them after the call with them that I would phone Tom Heidenberger and ask him if this was something he would like to do for his wife, Michele. I then phoned Tom and told him of the plan. He was so touched by it that he could not talk. I gave him all the time he needed. He finally got the energy to say thanks.

After my call with Tom Heidenberger, I received a call from Todd Wissing, who said he would put me in touch with the people who were in charge of honoring the flight crews at American and United Airlines.

OUR HEROES

It was one very difficult job putting together all those names of the flight crews. I had to make certain that all were spelled correctly, so I double- and triple-checked the names, all the time reading each name with the greatest respect, understanding that each of these names were heroes who died on September 11, 2001.

United Flight Crews from September 11th Tragedies

United Flight 175

Second plane to hit WTC
From Boston to Los Angeles
56 passengers

9 crew:
Victor Saracini, captain
Michael Horrocks, first officer
Robert J. Fangman, flight attendant
Amy N. Jarret, flight attendant
Amy R. King, flight attendant
Kathryn L. Yancey LaBorie, flight attendant
Alfred G. Marchand, flight attendant
Michael C. Tarrou, flight attendant
Alicia N. Titus, flight attendant

United Flight 93

Crashed in Somerset County, Pennsylvania
Boeing 757
From Newark, NJ to San Francisco
37 passengers

7 crew:
Jason Dahl, captain
LeRoy Homer, first officer
Lorraine G. Bay, flight attendant
Sandra W. Bradshaw, flight attendant
Wanda A. Green, flight attendant
CeeCee Lyles, flight attendant
Deborah A. Welsh, flight attendant

American Flight Crews from September 11th Tragedies

American Flight 11

First plane to hit WTC

Boeing 767

From Boston to Los Angeles

81 passengers

11 crew:

John Ogonowski, captain

Thomas McGuinness, first officer

Barbara Arestegui, flight attendant

Jeffrey Collman, flight attendant

Sara Low, flight attendant

Karen Martin, flight attendant

Kathleen Nicosia, flight attendant

Betty Ong, flight attendant

Jean Roger, flight attendant

Dianne Snyder, flight attendant

Madeline Sweeney, flight attendant

American Flight 77

Crashed into Pentagon

Boeing 757

From Washington's Dulles International Airport

to Los Angeles

58 Passengers

6 crew:

Charles Burlingame, captain

David Charlebois, first officer

Michele Heidenberger, flight attendant

Jennifer Lewis, flight attendant

Kenneth Lewis (Jennifer's husband), flight attendant

Renee May, flight attendant

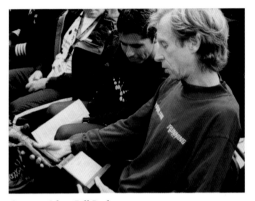

German Silva, Bill Rodgers

After making certain that my list of names was correct, I then had all the names engraved on a Fred Lebow statue replica that I planned to give to Captain Heidenberger, whose wife died on American Flight 77.

I also had an identical statue made for Mike Burr, which I would present at the ceremony at Dockweiler State Beach eight days after the Central Park dedication for Fred.

I also started putting together a list for the Dockweiler State Beach event that included California Lieutenant Governor Cruz Bustamante, Los Angeles Chief of Police Bernard Parks and his wife, Bobbie, Los Angeles City Councilman Tom LaBonge, and dear friend Bill Rodgers, who, when I told him about the event at the ceremony in New York, said he wanted to be there.

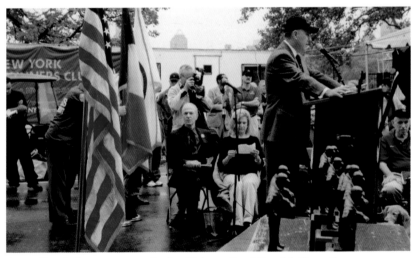

George Hirsch, Congresswoman Carolyn Maloney, Dan Mitrovich, Henry Stern

those services that are so badly needed at a time like this.

I also want to thank the Dale Carnegie organization, in particular J. Oliver Crom, Michael Crom, and his wife, Nancy, and my goddaughter Nicole, who are also with us here today.

In addition to them, I want to thank Peter Johnson and his wife, Brenda, who helped so much in preparing the event back on October 31, 1991.

My brother George, who served on our committee and helped with that original meeting in the Oval Office.

My dear friend Marjorie Martin and her friend, Mr. Terry Cook, a lead singer of the great Metropolitan Opera here in New York, who has agreed to sing today.

Scott Lange, who was originally hired by Fred Lebow to modernize the NYRRC and build the NYCMarathon in terms of sponsorship and marketing, became very important to me at the time as he is today as a go to person for advice. He was 100 percent in support of the statue of Fred.

There are a couple of people who could not be with us today. One is our honorary chairperson, US Senator Alan K. Simpson of Wyoming, who was so instrumental in opening the door to the White House and President George H.W. Bush.

Another is Congressman Jose Serrano, who serves the 15th District of New York. It was Congressman Serrano who paid tribute to Fred Lebow by entering into the Congressional Record of the 107th Congress, First Session, 'Tribute to the Permanent Endowment Ceremony of the Fred Lebow Statue: Founder of the New York City Marathon, on this day, Saturday, November 3, 2001.'

I personally want to thank Congressman Serrano for all his help and support of his friend Fred Lebow and for being a friend of mine.

I also want to recognize members of the New York Parks and Recreation, the Central Park Precinct of the New York Police Department, of which I once served as a member of the Auxiliary Police, and Tavern on the Green.

There are others to thank, but I will get to them later in the program.

Let me now introduce the Senior Minister to the Marble Collegiate Church here in New York City, the Reverend Dr. Arthur Caliandro, to do the invocation."

INVOCATION

"Will you bow your heads. Wondrous and loving God. We pause in this sacred moment to honor the memory of Fred Lebow, whose dream of a great marathon became a miraculous reality, the greatest marathon in the world.

Bless his memory and the continuing life of his dream. Lord, bless Dan Mitrovich, whose dream was the statue, and the sculptor, Jesus Dominguez, whose artistry made it a happening. And bless all who will run in this race tomorrow. We celebrate them, their discipline, their tenacity, and their dreams.

Keep them in loving care. Lord, we are a blessed people. We are grateful for so much. Thank you for your blessings and the blessing of this very special moment."

INTRODUCTION OF J. OLIVER CROM

At this time it is my pleasure to introduce a friend, not only to me but to all of us here today, and that is J. Oliver Crom, the CEO of Dale Carnegie.

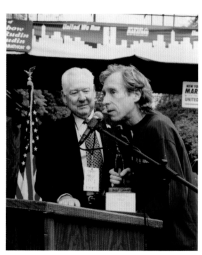

J. Oliver Crom in presentation of limited edition to Bill Rodgers

REMARKS BY MR. CROM

"Dan, as you all know and those who know him, is very generous with his accolades to us. But the person who really deserves accolades is Dan Mitrovich. Here is a man who had a vision, a vision of what could become.

He admired Fred Lebow because of what Fred established, not only because of the New York Marathon, but because of the qualities that Fred had. Because Fred was also a visionary, Fred was a man who respected perseverance, and if any person had vision in perseverance, it is Dan Mitrovich. At that Waldorf Astoria luncheon, we started eleven years ago, and I have to say that Dan Mitrovich is a salesman, but you all know that.

To think that out of that small seed that was planted, after eleven years we finally have the fulfillment of that dream, and that is the perseverance that Dan spoke of so many years ago. Dan has also given me the honor to present the first statue today to a recipient, and that person is Bill Rodgers."

J. OLIVER CROM PRESENTATION TO BILL RODGERS

"Frank Schroeder, Fred Lebow, and Bill Rodgers sparked the world's running boom. Your years of friendship with Fred Lebow, in respect for the accomplishment he brought to the running world, is known by all; therefore, your endorsement of the NYCMTC idea to honor Fred Lebow with a life-size statue here in New York Central Park was inevitable in obtaining the support of the running community."

—*J. Oliver Crom*

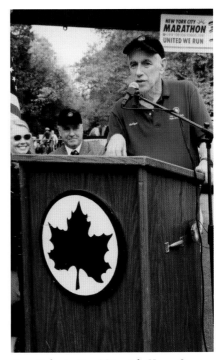

BILL RODGERS

"I remember when Fred got the statue, and I still look over to see the statue when I run through Central Park, and to me Fred is still here, the marathon is always going to be here, and Fred's spirit is celebrating with us today."

—*Bill Rodgers*

Anne Roberts, Dan Mitrovich, Henry Stern

REMARKS BY LEROY NEIMAN

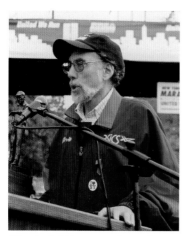

LeRoy Neiman

"Fred Lebow was a friend, and this modest piece of sculpture really reflects him, the skill of the man. He was a runner first, and that is how I remember him. In 1979 I did about three or four years of posters and so Fred and I had a meeting on it. When I finished it I gave Fred a call and told him I was finished.

'Do you want to look at it?' He was in his offices over on the east side. A few minutes later the phone rang from downstairs in the lobby, and it was Fred, he had run all the way over here to my place. His Road Runners cap was pulled over his head, he was in his sweatsuit, but he was not breathing very heavily.

He had kept his word and had run straight over to look at the painting.

This is what the man represents; he kept running and running, and a lot of things got done, and I am proud to have known him."

—*LeRoy Neiman*

PRESENTATION TO ALLAN STEINFELD

Allan Steinfeld receiving Limited Edition statue

"I am truly honored to receive this statue of Fred. It has my name on it, but it obviously belongs to our staff and our board that backs us and makes this race happen. I have told people I am an orchestra leader, and I am, but I have great instruments to work with. I can't play an instrument, but I got a wonderful team to work with.

Fred was there greeting the winners when they came across the finish line, but he was also out there to greet the average runner, and it is the average runners who remember Fred being out there hours and hours, cheering them on. He created an event that is, of course, a world class event, but it is a people's event. This race is about people and it is about vision, Fred's vision."

—*Allan Steinfeld*

BERNIE COOPER PRESENTATION TO GEORGE HIRSCH

"There are many people in many ways who contributed to this marvelous sport, and we are all here to honor one of them, the publisher of *Runner's World* magazine, a magazine that really took this beginning activity and helped broker it up into a massive enterprise of runners and races all over the world. It is my pleasure to introduce George Hirsch."

ACCEPTANCE BY GEORGE HIRSCH

"I am delighted to be here for this incredible tribute to Fred, a great friend of all of ours."

—*George Hirsch*

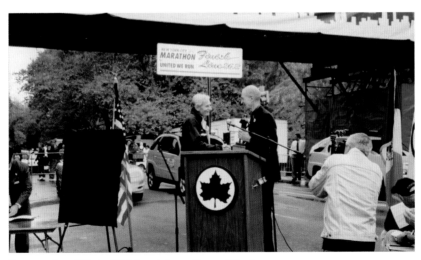

Presentation of Limited Edition statue to George Hirsch

MICHAEL CROM, NOVEMBER 3, 2001

"At Dale Carnegie we like to recognize individuals who show great vision. As a company that was founded here in New York City back in 1912 at 112th Street, we feel that Fred Lebow has recognized the true vision of New York. It was our honor to be involved from the very beginning and we recognize that vision."

—Michael Crom

INTRODUCTION OF GRETE WAITZ BY BERNIE COOPER

"It is my privilege to introduce the winner of nine New York City Marathons and, as Allan Steinfeld reminded me, the tenth, which she ran with Fred Lebow, was the very best that she ran. It is a real privilege to introduce a friend of mine and extraordinary person in the field of running, Grete Waitz."

ACCEPTANCE BY GRETE WAITZ

"It is a great honor to receive Fred's statue. Fred touched a lot of lives, mine in a big way. What would Grete Waitz do today if it wasn't for Fred Lebow? I probably would have ended my running career on the track and in cross country, but I came, as Fred was very gracious and invited me. I came and I won and thought that was it, as when I finished, I said never, never am I going to ever do this again. But I turned into a marathon runner and had a wonderful career for ten more years, and then Fred and I, until my last competitive race in 1990.

And that was all because of Fred, and then I ran with Fred in 1992, and I know that Fred always wanted me to get my tenth marathon victory, but I can assure you that crossing that finish line in five and a half hours was so much more than winning a tenth marathon. I owe a lot to Fred, and I am proud and honored to get this statue of him today."

—Grete Waitz

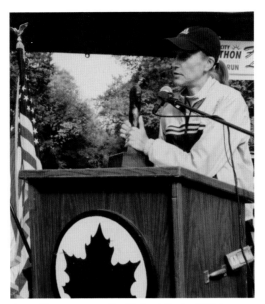

Grete Waitz receiving Fred Lebow Limited Edition statue

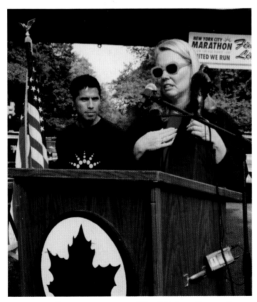

German Silva presentation of Fred Lebow Limited Edition statue to Anne Roberts

INTRODUCTION OF GERMAN SILVA

"To give the next presentation, I want to introduce the winner of both the 1994 and 1995 New York City Marathons, German Silva."

INTRODUCTION OF ANN ROBERTS BY GERMAN SILVA

"It is with great pleasure that I have this opportunity to present the Fred Lebow statue to my very dear friend and the woman who was so close to Fred, Ms. Anne Roberts."

ACCEPTANCE BY ANN ROBERTS

"Thank you, German. I was going to spare you a speech, but German wanted me to say something, and I just want everyone to know that Fred was more than just about this race, he was the most special, bravest, kindest man I have ever known.

Thank you Dan and Linda."

—*Anne Roberts*

INTRODUCTION OF CAROLYN MALONEY

"It is with great pleasure that I now introduce our next recipient of the Fred Lebow statue. It was her early support back in 1994 that helped make possible this permanent placement today of the Fred Lebow statue.

She is a marvelous woman with great passion for things she believes in, and Fred Lebow had the great pleasure of having her believe in him.

I now introduce New York 12th District Congresswoman Carolyn Maloney."

REMARKS BY CAROLYN MALONEY

"Thank you so much, Dan, and your family, and Mr. Crom, and all your team who turned your vision and idea into the reality of this wonderful statue and this living legacy that we will all enjoy for many, many years

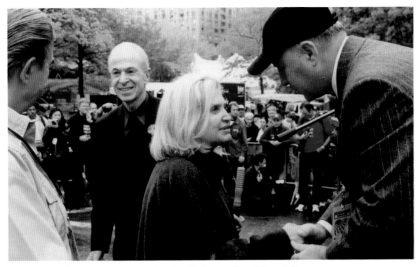

George Hirsch, Congresswoman Carolyn Maloney, Dan Mitrovich

to come. On behalf of all our marathon runners, of whom my husband is one, we particularly say thank you. The marathon has been part of our life since 1976 when it became a citywide marathon, and it is a great celebration of which we can all participate. Whether you are running, or cheering people on, or volunteering, it is one of the great events in New York, and it exemplifies a celebration of bringing us all together.

Earlier on, Dan mentioned September 11. I don't think it is ever far from our minds, and I couldn't help but think about our event when he was speaking, and I thought the real difference between our country and Americans and the terrorists is that the terrorists destroyed and wanted to destroy people who were different from them, whereas in our country we celebrate our differences, and we celebrate our democracy that welcomes so many people to be part of our country. As we run tomorrow and celebrate our marathon, we will have at least one hundred different nationalities, and thank you so much for making this happen. Thank you for bringing this reality to all of us to enjoy, and if you ever think that one person can't make a difference, look to the life of Fred Lebow and what he meant to all of us and will continue to mean to so many people."

—*Carolyn Maloney*

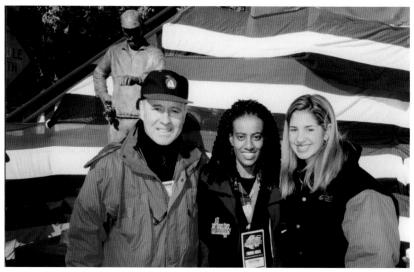

Dan Mitrovich, Daughter of Abebe Bikila, Tsige Abebe, Marissa Mitrovich

REMARKS BY HENRY STERN

"On September 13, 1970, we had 127 participants. In 1976 we expanded to all five boroughs, and for this we thank Fred Lebow.

The image of him in his trademark suit that he used to wear, and his pose, will inspire generations of runners.

I want to close by making one comparison.

A vision is an obsession that succeeds, just like revolution is treason that succeeds, and here we have two men, similar in the fact that they both had obsessions. Fred was to create the New York City Marathon, and through thirty years of work he did it and made it wonderful. It was copied all over the country and all over the world. He is the principal figure of the growth of twentieth century marathoning as a public sport, which is an extraordinary accomplishment meriting this statue, apart from his qualities of character.

Daniel Mitrovich had a different vision. He wanted to make a statue of Fred Lebow, so, as Boswell described the works of Samuel Johnson, he held to his vision. It took him eleven years, crossing the continent many times, dealing with different mayors and public officials. He succeeded, and that's why his contribution will be permanent and will be recognized in a historical sign that we will write and affix to the Lebow monument. So I am so pleased that Daniel has lived to see the day the statue is done, and that I am still commissioner. I have been commissioner fifteen years now, seven years under Mayor Koch, then I was fired, and eight years under Giuliani. Now there is an election on Tuesday, and I may be fired again, that's all right.

What's nice is that this glorious event, eleven years in the making, happened on my watch, and I am enormously proud to have had this chance to thank Daniel and salute Fred's memory."

—*Henry Stern*

REMARKS BY BOBBY BARRETT

"My name is Bobby Barrett, and I serve as General Vice Chairman to a 350-member tribe of the Viejas Band of Kumeyaay Indians. We are small

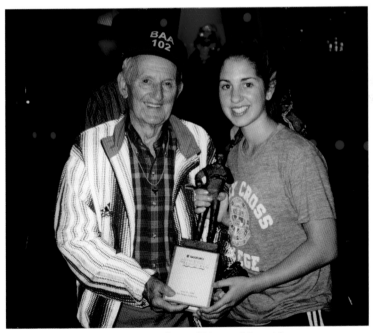

Boston Marathon legend Johnny Kelley and Marissa Mitrovich

but very, very proud to be here today. We have all become New Yorkers in our hearts since September 11th.

I have come to know Fred. That Fred stood for freedom, kindness, and spirit. I have come to know his love for his people. His love for his running but, most of all, his love for people running. God bless America and God bless New York City."

—*Bobby Barrett*

REMARKS BY TOM HEIDENBERGER

"Members of the tribute committee, honored guests, ladies and gentlemen, I am honored to be standing before you today on behalf of my wife, Michelle, and the rest of the airline employees lost on September 11th, honoring the Fred Lebow statue and all that Fred stood for.

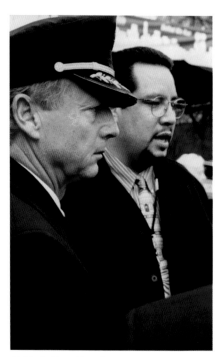

Bobby L. Barrett and Captain Tom Heidenberger

The air crews of the flights on September 11, as it turns out, are also uniting a nation. My wife Michelle's name is on this miniature statue, but along with her name are the names of many other true American heroes. They live, doing their jobs, living their lives with excellence and grace, and that is also how they died. Whether flying the aircraft, insuring the safety of the passengers, or simply smiling their smiles, laughing their laughs, they epitomize the one thing in this country that we always said we hold dear: the American way of life. That is something we, because of their sacrifice, now treasure more than ever. I am

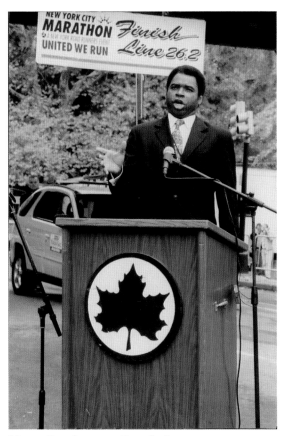

Metropolitan Opera star Terry Cook

proud of my profession and the professionals who responded to the crippling blow this country suffered with confidence and bravery. When the country was paralyzed, the nation's eyes turned to the airline crews, and they put aside their fears and did what the country needed them to do, and they got back in the air. Michelle and the rest of the brave heroes of September 11th will stand for all time as pioneers who led this country back to the determined routes that let us rise to greatness as a nation. We look at September 11, a day that will live in infamy forever. As we see how this life has changed, we also remember that it is important that our way of life remains the same and we do the things we need to do to protect it. The people's names that appear on this statue are depending on us to do that. Because of the heroes of Flights 11, 93, 77, and 175, we are now the Reunited States of America and we will only grow stronger in our resolve. Thank you!"

—*Tom Heidenberger, Captain US Airways*

"I will now read the names of flight crews of American Flights 11 and 77, and United Flights 93 and 177, to be followed by Mr. Terry Cook of the New York Metropolitan Opera singing 'God Bless America.'

On Friday, November 16, 2001, *The Daily Plant,* a newspaper published by the New York City Department of Parks and Recreation said:

'At a dedication ceremony on Saturday, November 3, one day before the race, Commissioner Henry J. Stern accepted the statue of Fred Lebow into the Parks' collection of monuments. With that, Lebow joined the ranks of Shakespeare, Hans Christian Anderson, and Duke Ellington, all of whom are figured in the park. The image of Lebow, posed checking his watch, will inspire generations of runners and remind them of the man who did so much to popularize their sport.'"

Following the event, some officials of American Airlines, along with Bobby Barrett and Ral Christman, were taken to Ground Zero by the Commander of the Parks Police.

Ral Christman performed a sacred ceremony in honor of those who had perished there. Both men told me later that it was one of the most emotional moments they had ever experienced. They told me that the police, who ushered them through four checkpoints, cried as they shared their memories of what had happened on 9/11. Bobby, who went on to become Tribal Chairman, told me he still thinks about that day and that every time he goes into the Viejas Tribal offices, he takes a moment to look at the statue of Fred Lebow.

After the beautiful event in Central Park, we found ourselves a week later at the beach at the end of the Los Angeles International Airport to finalize the Americans United Flag Across America.

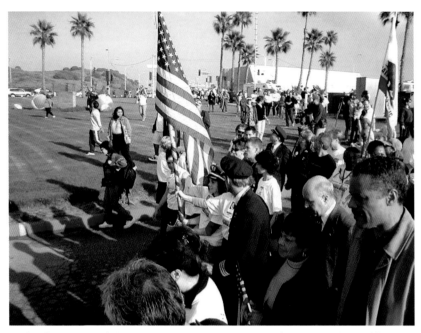

Dockweiler State Beach Ceremony, 11/11/2001. American Airlines First Officer Todd Wissing, Daniel S. Mitrovich, Mrs. Bobby Parks, Los Angeles Chief of Police Bernard Parks

Prior to the event starting at Dockweiler, more than seventy family members of the crews and passengers who lost their lives walked around the horseshoe loop of LAX and under the tunnel on Sepulveda, then headed down Imperial Highway, west toward Dockweiler State Beach. At the beach family members were greeted by a reception crowd of more than five hundred people. The program began with Tucker Fleming's playing of the bagpipes, presentation of colors by the United States Marine Color Guard, and the National Anthem sung by Ms. Beth Gray.

The program continued with Todd Wissing, First Officer, American Airlines, who served as National Communications Coordinator, welcoming everyone to Dockweiler. Todd Wissing then introduced Los Angeles Police Chief Bernard Parks, who welcomed everyone to Los Angeles. Chief Parks talked about the role that the police played in New York and how difficult an assignment it was, knowing how many of their colleagues had died on that horrific day in New York. He spoke of how many of the LAPD force volunteered to help in New York and how proud he was of his fellow police officers.

After Chief Parks spoke, Todd Wissing introduced Mike Burr, National Director of Americans United Flag Across America. I was then introduced, along with Bill Rodgers, to present to Mike Burr the Fred Lebow statue replica, showing the names of the flight crews engraved on that replica.

Todd Wissing introduced Lt. Governor Cruz Bustamante, who gave a moving speech in which he said that, "Today, we begin to heal as a nation. Today we are a United America."

The program ended with the singing of "God Bless America" by Ms. Autumn Carlson, daughter of American Airlines Captain Don Carlson.

City of New York
Parks & Recreation

The Arsenal
Central Park
New York, New York 10021

Henry J. Stern
Commissioner

6 Dec 01

Mr. Daniel Mitrovich
619 Kettner Boulevard
San Diego, CA 92101

Statue Man

Dear Mr. Mitrovich:

Thank you for organizing the endowment for the Fred Lebow Statue and the dedication ceremony. It was a lovely event.

We are pleased that you and the New York City Marathon Committee were committed to realizing the creation of the Fred Lebow statue and ensuring its permanent home in Central Park. The ceremony was a nice homage to Fred Lebow and those dedicated to the New York Marathon. Sunday was a perfect day for the run and we were pleased to see so many people participate, including several Parkies.

I hope that you will visit New York often to see the statue at its new home at Runner's Gate and again next November when it is brought to the finish line to inspire runners from around the world. Enjoy the enclosed photographs from the event. Should you have any questions, please call me at (212) 360-1305.

All the best,

Star Quest

Henry J. Stern

November 6, 2001

Mr. Daniel S. Mitrovich
President and Founder
New York City Marathon Tribute
   Committee

Dear Dan:

I am pleased to extend my congratulations to you and
to all the members of the New York City Marathon
Tribute Committee on the permanent endowment of the
Fred Lebow memorial in Central Park.

Every athletic competition has the potential to bring
out the best in us. As we strive to develop our
skills, we find untapped energy and talent. When we
finally put our training to the test, we join with
dedicated individuals who share our enthusiasm for
friendly competition.

For more than 30 years, the New York City Marathon
has epitomized this fine tradition, and it is fitting
that its founder, Fred Lebow, should be remembered in
this meaningful way. The Fred Lebow statue will
stand as a shining symbol of all that we cherish
about the Marathon and of the values to which Fred
dedicated his life: the spirit of teamwork, the
ideal of sportsmanship, the solidarity of a city, and
the commitment to personal excellence that is shared
by athletes around the world.

I thank all those whose hard work, vision, and
perseverance brought this memorial to reality and
send my best wishes for the future.

Sincerely,

Bill Clinton

Congressional Record

United States of America

PROCEEDINGS AND DEBATES OF THE *107th* CONGRESS, FIRST SESSION

House of Representatives

Tribute to the Permanent Endowment Ceremony of the Fred Lebow Statue: Founder of New York City Marathon

HON. JOSÉ E. SERRANO
OF NEW YORK

Saturday, November 3, 2001

Mr. Speaker, it is with joy and pride that I rise today to pay tribute to the permanent endowment ceremony of the Fred Lebow monument, to honor the late founder of the great New York City Marathon, the world's greatest marathon which will take place on November 4, 2001.

Seven years ago, Mr. Daniel S. Mitrovich spearheaded the effort to honor Fred Lebow, founder of the New York City Marathon, by erecting a statue of the visionary athlete. I was honored to have been a part of the monumental event that commemorated the creator of this great race. Fred Lebow, as Director of the New York City Road Runners Club, Inc., founded the marathon and nurtured it from a 126-runner race to one of the largest and most well-known marathons in the world. This year, the grand monument will be waiting at the finish line to greet weary runners and will later find a permanent home at the 67th Street entrance to Central Park, fulfilling the promise Mr. Mitrovich made 10 years ago when he said that he would ensure that a statue of Fred Lebow would someday stand in Central Park.

Mr. Speaker, I am grateful for the continued dedication of the New York Road Runners Club, Inc. and the New York City Marathon Tribute Committee. Their work is essential to maintaining the spirit of the New York City Marathon and helps fuel the great spirit of the city itself. The New York City Marathon has never been more important than it will be this year. Organized under the theme "United We Stand," this race of endurance and power represents the will and essence of the city, New Yorkers, Americans, and of peace-loving people all over the world. We are all indebted to Mr. Lebow, who lost his battle with brain cancer on October 9, 1994, for organizing and fostering a great athletic and humanitarian event and the permanent endowment of his likeness in Central Park is fitting and worthy of celebration. Also, as proof of his accomplishments, Mr. Lebow was inducted in the 2001 National Distance Running Hall of Fame.

The New York City Marathon has united people across all walks of life since its inception 31 years ago because it is both a test of perseverance and a celebration of life. Runners vary in athletic ability, age, race and religion but share a common desire to run New York City. This year, runners will share something else as well. They will share an understanding that they are integral parts of New York's resurrecting spirit and perhaps that knowledge will energize flagging feet as they cover the great length of New York City. The sense of unity among the human family will be invincible when over 30,000 runners from around the world join in New York City to bond with it as only runners can do.

I ask my colleagues to join me in honoring Fred Lebow's life achievements and the permanent endowment of his statue in Central Park, as well as commending the continued efforts of Daniel Mitrovich to preserve the integrity and excellence of the New York City Marathon.

18

BOSTON STRONG 117

"I often went to Fred for advice and counsel that he freely gave me. Whatever Fred did, he knew in his heart that it was the right thing to do for the Marathon."

—Guy Morse, Director, Boston Marathon

MONDAY APRIL 15, 2013, PATRIOTS DAY in Boston … Ethiopian runner Lelisa Desisa ended the dominance of the Kenyans, winning the Boston Marathon with a time of 2:10:22.

After three straight victories, the Kenyan winning streak was over for the men. However, Kenyan Rita Jeptoo won the Women's Division in a time of 2:26:25, for her second Boston Marathon victory, her first being in 2006.

Unfortunately, that was not the story that we all remember about the 117th running of the Boston Marathon. One hour, fifty-nine minutes after Lelisa Desisa crossed the finish line, a bomb exploded near the finish line, and then a second bomb went off, some fifteen seconds later, not far from where the runners make the final turn onto Boylston Street from Hereford Street.

This tragic event struck terror in Boston, killing three at and near the finish line and injuring 264 people. Most of the people injured were just people watching the race, cheering on the runners, friends and family of this great marathon.

On Thursday evening at about 10:30 p.m., the same two terrorists also assassinated MIT police officer Sean Collier in what was described by the media as a cold-blooded ambush.

Officer Collier was to be laid to rest in Puritan Lawn Memorial Park, Peabody, Essex County, Massachusetts.

On Wednesday, April 24, 2013, a memorial service was held in Cambridge which was attended by Vice President Joe Biden and his wife, Dr. Jill Biden. The vice president called the brothers accused of killing Collier and detonating the Boston Marathon blast, "Two twisted, perverted, cowardly, knock-off jihadis."

I personally know of Dr. Biden's total dedication to her running and of her respect for runners. (U.S. Marine Corps Marathon 1998-4:30:02.) Dr. Biden stopped by an area where fresh concrete was poured into a spot where one of the blasts occurred. She left flowers and placed a pair of running shoes.

One of the 264 injured was Richard "Dick" Donohue Jr., a thirty-three-year-old police officer for the Massachusetts Bay Transportation Authority, who was responding to a call Friday morning to assist Sean Collier. When Officer Donohue got out of his car, he exchanged

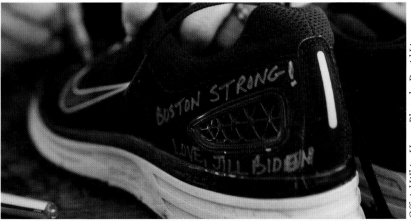

Dr. Jill Biden's running shoes

gunfire with the two suspected terrorists who had just gunned down Sean Collier.

Officer Donohue survived.

Eight-year-old Dorchester resident Martin Richard, twenty-nine-year-old Krystle Campbell of Medford, Massachusetts, and twenty-three-year-old Boston University graduate student from China, Lu Lingzi, were also murdered by the two terrorists. I will not list the names of the two terrorists, as they do not belong in the same book as the three they murdered.

Martin, Krystle, and Lu were just having fun, cheering on the runners, not hurting anyone, letting life be life, and yet two, sick, horrible monsters took their precious lives away from them and from all who knew and loved them.

I remember so well crossing the finish line five times in the Boston Marathon, and each of those five times was one of the most special times of my life. I remember my wife, Linda, waiting for me at that finish line in three of those races. She not only cheered me on, but she cheered all the runners. Being at the finish line of a marathon is one of her most favorite things to do in life.

To the families and to all the spectators at marathons, we, the runners, appreciate you so much. The millions of people who cheer on marathon runners all over the world are just wonderful people, often giving hope to the runners that they can finish, and showing just how proud they are of the hard work that each of us runners put into in training for a 26.2 mile event.

I remember the day before the big race in 1996 for the one hundredth anniversary of the Boston Marathon. Several days before, when I was flying from San Diego to Boston, the idea came to me to arrange to have all the runners from San Diego attend a photo op at the finish line of the Boston Marathon the day before the race was run.

Three hundred twenty-one runners from San Diego were running the Boston Marathon that year, and many of them showed up for that photo. I had made a large sign for the photo op which I held up at the finish line, hoping that runners would show up and, yes, they did. They came from every direction. I think we had more than 150 runners from San Diego show up for that photo. After the marathon I had each of the 321 names engraved on a plaque. I then wrote a brief story, and along with my 100th Boston Marathon Medal and the photo of that day, I had it beautifully framed, and I presented it to the Hall of Champions in San Diego, where it hangs today.

Linda and I were at our office when we received two text messages from our two sons, Jesse and Luke, telling of this bomb explosion at the finish line of the marathon.

Both Linda and I were just sick about this despicable, horrible tragedy. We just collapsed in our chairs behind our desks. We have so much love

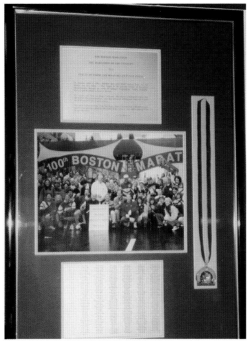

Framed picture given to the Hall of Champions in San Diego by Dan Mitrovich who framed his 100th Boston Marathon medal and had each runner from San Diego's name engraved along with a photo of many of those participants.

for that marathon. It is so much a part of our life of so many good times, good friends, and good stories.

I jumped on the Internet to read as much as I could about what had just happened in Boston. First, I called Anne Roberts to see if, by chance, she was in Boston, and then I called Allan Steinfeld. Anne answered and told me she was not in Boston but in New York, but many of her friends were there in Boston.

I reached Allan, who was in lockdown in the Copley Square Hotel. We talked about the senseless bombing that just took place, and at the time of the call, we still had no news if there were others involved.

After the calls to Anne and Allan, I sat at my desk, just numb. *How sad, how tragic*, kept going over and over in my mind.

I started receiving text messages from a number of people, as well as friends who knew of Linda's and my involvement in marathons. They all thought we might have been there.

On Wednesday I looked at the faces of Martin Richard and Krystle Campbell that appeared in photos published by the *Los Angeles Times*. When I looked at those photos, it made me so sad. How can someone be so evil as to eliminate from our world two of these gorgeous human beings?

On Thursday I read a story in the *Los Angeles Times* about a grad student attending Boston University, Chinese victim Lu Lingzi, which again caused me to pause and say a prayer for this international student who came to America to study and now, on account of two terrorists, was dead.

That evening Linda and our daughter Heidi were waiting to be seated at one of our favorite Mexican restaurants, Pacos, in West Los Angeles. A young lady and her boyfriend were seated next to us and asked me about the running shoes I was wearing.

We found out that we all had a lot in common—marathoning. My total of ten was pale compared to both of their totals. She had run eighteen and her boyfriend thirty total marathons, to date.

We started talking about the bombing in Boston, and she said that many of her friends said she should stop doing marathons on account of the bombing. And then she said the following:

"What happened Monday is so awfully horrible, but we can't be scared to live life. We can't hide. We live in a free society, and that makes us vulnerable, sometimes. We can't hole up in our homes. We still get to go to the mall, concerts, and outdoor weddings without fear. This won't stop me from running. I might even run harder. I love marathons and I won't let this tragedy take away my happiness.

I will continue to run marathons and this bombing will not stop me!"

The next day in my office, my staff person, Maira, brought in a picture that someone had just tweeted to my blog. The tweet was a photo of the Fred Lebow statue in Central Park, but this time Fred was wearing a runner's jacket, and it was not just a runner's jacket but a Boston Marathon jacket.

Also attached to the statue were two signs, one reading: "I run for Boston," and the other which said, "As our hearts cry, our legs are growing stronger." Also, a runner had placed flowers in Fred's hand.

This person had felt so bad about the Boston incident that she decided to do what made her feel better, and that was to go for a run over to the Fred Lebow statue and place this Boston Marathon jacket on Fred.

She knew how sad Fred would have been about this horrible event, and she was right. Had Fred been alive, he would have been in Boston and may well have been near the finish line.

Fred loved to see runners crossing the finish line, as

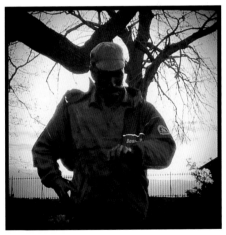

Fred Lebow statue in Boston Strong track jacket

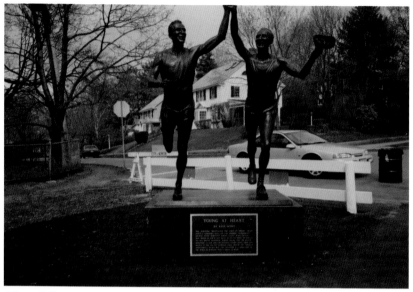

Johnny Kelley Statue, Young at Heart by Rich Muno (1993)

each and every runner who crosses the finish line has a different story about why they are running. Runners are special people.

As I think of Fred, I cannot help but think of the legendary Boston Marathon runner Johnny Kelley, who passed away at the age of ninety-seven. Johnny Kelley completed his first Boston Marathon in 1933. He won it in 1935 and 1945. He finished in the top ten eighteen times and fifteen times in the top five.

Johnny Kelley would have cried a lot of tears for those who lost their lives, for the spectators who were injured, and for his race, the Boston Marathon.

If you are ever in Boston, you need to go to "Heartbreak Hill" in Newton, Massachusetts, at the corner of Walnut Street and Commonwealth Avenue, and there you will see the statue of Johnny Kelley titled: "Young at Heart." By sculptor Rich Muno, the sculpture depicts Johnny in his racing days when he was twenty, grasping the hand of another figure of himself as a running octogenarian.

Johnny Kelley ran in sixty-one Boston Marathons and finished in fifty-eight of them. Johnny Kelley was a hero of Dennis, Massachusetts.

Each year in his honor, there is a Johnny Kelley Half Marathon. Also, the town honored Johnny with a park in his name.

Thinking of Fred and Johnny at this time makes me think of none other than "Boston Billy" Bill Rodgers, who ran a total of seventeen times in the Boston Marathon. As I have said in a previous chapter, he won four times: 1975, 1978, 1979, and 1980. He also won New York Marathons four times. Twenty-eight of his marathon times were under 2:15. Altogether, he won a total of twenty-two marathons!

In an interview with writer Josh Levin of the Slate Group, Rodgers said on Tuesday, April 16, 2013, that, "Monday's attack transformed that nexus of celebration into a crime scene."

But Rodgers believes that nobody can change what this race stands for. In *Marathon Man*, Rodgers' autobiography, he writes about how powerful it felt to run through the Boston crowd. "As the miles wore on, their support for me was a tangible thing that hung in the air. Their cheers continually charged me up like a battery, inspiring me to push even harder, to succeed even more." But this wasn't because Rodgers was a champion and a hometown kid. "I think this is true for everyone who runs Boston," he writes. "The crowd's support lifts them up." Boston Billy vows that he'll be back at the marathon that gave him his name, as the race's biggest supporter, if no longer a competitive runner. "All my friends are going to run next year," he says. "Are you kidding me? They would never ever let those puny people treat us that way and get away with it. They won't get away with it. They Won't Get Away With It."

A FINAL NOTE

The Boston bomber was found guilty on all thirty counts on April 8, 2015.

He was sentenced to death on May 17, 2015. The jury deliberated for over fourteen hours, which brings to a close for most of us, but not all of us, these horrible, senseless killings that happened on April 15, 2013.

As Billy Rodgers said, "They won't get away with it," and they didn't!

Epilogue
FOREVER AT THE FINISH LINE

A S I SPEAK TO YOU, THE reader, I first want you to know how much I appreciate you buying my book, taking the time to read it, and now having a better understanding of why I wrote it in the first place.

I'm sorry that it took me so long to write, as many of the wonderful people I talk about in this book have passed on in life.

Grete Waitz, George Plimpton, Dr. Arthur Caliandro, Warner LeRoy, Marjorie Martin, LeRoy Neiman, Bernard J. Cooper, Johnny Kelley, and Alberto Arroyo, the Mayor of Central Park, to name a few.

In life we are blessed if we have a story to write, like I have been with *Forever at the Finish Line*. It was Fred's gift to me.

Fred gave me an incredible opportunity that has blessed my life since 1990. To be able to know a man like Fred in one's lifetime is a wonderful gift to me.

It has always been my belief that people who have accomplished so much, for so many, and were so unselfish in their way of going about it, deserve to have someone say something nice about it.

Henry Stern said, "I only hope that when I die, I have someone like Dan Mitrovich to tell about my life."

When I heard those words, I felt so blessed and loved, all at the same time. Thank you, Henry!

This book may have my name on the cover, but the ones written about inside are the true writers of *Forever at the Finish Line*, for without them there would be no book.

When you have an idea and you want to accomplish it, it will always be important to have people at your side. My wife, Linda, is one of those people. She, her giving of her time, and her passion that have helped me fulfill my dream, have blessed me!

Sincerely,
Daniel S. Mitrovich

Certificate
Of
Transfer of Ownership

The New York City Marathon Tribute Committee, a California Non-Profit Committee No. 33-063-6922, hereby transfers ownership of the Life-Size Bronze Statue of Fred Lebow by artist Jesus Dominguez, "Forever at the Finish Line," to the City of New York Department of Parks and Recreation.

Dated this 3rd Day of November in the year 2001.

Signatures below signify the right to transfer said ownership.

_____
Daniel S. Mitrovich
President and Founder

_____
Steve Scott
Board of Directors

_____
Anne Roberts
Board of Directors

_____
Dr. Keith Jeffery
Board of Directors

FRED LEBOW STATUE
Central Park

This life-sized bronze sculpture depicts Fred Lebow (1932–1994), who is best remembered as the founder of the world-renowned New York City Marathon and longtime president of the New York Road Runners Club. The sculpture was created by Jesus Ygnacio Dominguez and shows Lebow in his trademark running suit and hat, checking his watch as runners cross the finish line.

The sixth of seven children, Lebow was born Fischel Lebowitz in Arad, Romania on June 3, 1932. In his youth he hid from the Nazis and later fled from the Communists, making brief stops in England, Ireland, Czechoslovakia and other European countries before settling in the United States. After moving to New York City, Lebow embarked on a successful career in the garment and textile industry.

Lebow began running to improve his stamina for tennis, but soon realized that running was his true passion. In 1970 he organized the first New York City Marathon, which was run entirely in Central Park with only 127 participants. Lebow used his own money to purchase prizes for the first ten people to cross the finish line. In 1976 the Marathon was re-routed to travel through the streets of all five of New York's boroughs. The race now attracts more than 30,000 runners each year, and is supported by major corporate sponsors.

Lebow envisioned the New York City Marathon as a race for everyone — men and women of every color, creed and country, regardless of ability. Each runner seeks his or her own goal — whether to win, to achieve a personal best, or simply to finish.

Lebow served as president of the New York Road Runners club from 1972 until his retirement in 1993, after which he was feted by Mayor Giuliani at a Gracie Mansion reception. Under Lebow's direction the NYRRC instituted programs and events which popularized running and helped provide a safe atmosphere in Central Park. The NYRRC flourished and became the largest running club in the world.

Lebow was diagnosed with brain cancer in 1990. He ran his final marathon in 1992 with Grete Waitz in celebration of his 60th birthday and his cancer's temporary remission. Lebow finally succumbed to cancer on October 9, 1994.

To honor Lebow's vision and work Daniel Mitrovich created the New York City Marathon Tribute Committee and commissioned this sculpture. It was unveiled November 4, 1994 in a ceremony held near the Marathon's finish line near the West Drive at 67th Street in Central Park. The event was attended by 23 former winners of the New York City Marathon, Mr. Lebow's family and friends, and hundreds of running enthusiasts. On November 1, 2001 the sculpture was reinstalled on a new black granite pedestal at 90th Street and the East Drive in Central Park, where runners gather daily to work out together. For the Marathon each year, the Lebow statue returns to a spot within view of the finish line amidst the cheering spectators.

City of New York
Parks & Recreation

Rudolph W. Giuliani, Mayor
Henry J. Stern, Commissioner

November 2001

"FOREVER AT THE FINISH LINE"
STATUE HISTORY

November 4, 1990   Daniel S. Mitrovich, a runner from California, runs the New York City Marathon

January 31, 1991   Fred Lebow is honored in the Oval Office by President George Bush. Also in attendance are Senator Alan K. Simpson, Daniel S. Mitrovich, and George Mitrovich.

March 1, 1991   Daniel S. Mitrovich conceives the idea to honor Fred Lebow with a life-size statue.

October 31, 1991   Grete Waitz unveils the maquette and presents it to Fred on behalf of the New York City Marathon Tribute Committee at a luncheon undersritten by Dale Carnegie & Associates.

October 24, 1994   Continental Airlines flies statue to NYC.

Novermber 4, 1994   Statue unveiled at the New York City Marathon finish line in Central Park.

November 6, 1994   Statue placed in storage.

March 1, 1995   Statue flown to Los Angeles for the 10th Annual LA Marathon

March 4, 1995   Statue exhibited in Los Angeles.

March 5, 1995   Statue lost somewhere in Los Angeles.

March 7, 1995   Statue found locked in a truck somewhere in Los Angeles.

March 10, 1995   Statue returned to NYC and stored in a warehouse.

June 27, 1995   Statue placed at Tavern on the Green across from New York City Marathon finish line under a temporary permit.

October 27, 1995	The first of 100 bronze statue replicas presented to President Clinton at a White House ceremony.
November 3, 2001	Fred Lebow statue ceremony honoring the permamnent placement in Central Park.
November 5, 2001	Statue moves to its permanent location at 90th and 5th Avenue in New York City.

CREDITS

PHOTO CREDITS

Official White House Photographer

Sharon Farmer

Marathon Foto

San Diego Union-Tribune

Ken Levinson, Photographer

George Plimpton

Achilles Track Club International

British Pathé

San Diego Marathon (1981) Official Photographer

ECVHS 1960 Yearbook Photographer

1990 New York Marathon Photographer

Siphotos

Courtesy Santa Monica Track Club

Virginia Walk of Fame

Southcoast Air Quality Photo

YS Media.Com

Photo Run.net

David Gutierrez

New York Parks Department

Daniel S. Mitrovich

Dale Carnegie

New York Road Runners Club

Wikimedia Commons

YouTube.com

New York Times

PEOPLE INTERVIEWED FOR THIS BOOK

Michael Crom

Anne Roberts

Estee Stimler

Sara Katz

Henry Stern

Guy Morse

John Tope

Jesus Ygnacio Dominguez

George Hirsch

George Mitrovich

Marissa Mitrovich

Linda Mitrovich

Allan Steinfeld

Steve Scott

RESOURCES/PUBLICATIONS

New York Times
Runner's World
Rodale Press
New York Daily News
Boston Globe
New York Road Runners Club
Los Angeles Times
San Diego Union Tribune
Central Park Conservancy
Anything For A T-Shirt - Syracuse University Press
Go Achilles! by Dick Traum and Mary Bryant, edited by Megan
    Wynne-Lombardo
The Braemar Royal Highland Society
Stories To Tell Books
J. Oliver Crom

Index

144, 147, 148, 150, 156, 168,
169, 173, 176, 177, 178, 179,
181, 182, 183, 184, 185, 186,
188, 189, 190, 191, 192, 194,
200, 206, 207
Lennon, John, 80
Leone, Giacoma, 152
LeRoy, Jennifer Oz, 137
LeRoy, Mervyn, 137
LeRoy, Warner L., 121, 135, 136, 137,
208
Levin, John, 207
Levinson, Ken, 121
Lewis, Carl, 90, 91
Lewis, Steve, 91
Library of Congress, 42
Lincoln Memorial, 42
Lingzi, Lu, 202, 204
Longfellow Bridge, 60
Loroupe, Tegla, 93, 94, 128, 152
Louis, Spiridon, 34

M

McCain, John, 100
McColgan, Liz, 124
McDew, Darren W., 158
McGrath, Frank, 180
Madison Avenue Bridge, 16
Mahle, C. Emmett, 71, 74
Maloney, Carolyn, 178, 188, 189
Marble Collegiate Church, 32, 178, 181
Marcus Garvey Park, 17
Martin, Elliot, 11, 177
Martin, Marjorie, 11, 177, 178, 181, 208
Massachusetts Institute of Technology
(MIT), 60
Mattiessen, Peter, 88
Mayer, Raleigh, 102, 121, 134
Meston, W.A., 40
Meyer, Greg, 97
Minuet, Peter, 79
Mishima, Keizo, 121

Mitrovich, Bill, 36, 43, 44
Mitrovich, Daniel, 9, 24, 25, 28, 31,
32,33, 49, 50, 52, 73, 74, 82, 84,
116, 125, 134, 135, 138, 157,
168, 182, 183, 188, 189, 190,
191, 209
Mitrovich, George 21, 24, 25, 28, 51,
48, 63, 68, 69, 90, 95, 100, 103,
125, 156, 158, 180, 181
Mitrovich, Linda Brannon, 32, 61,
64, 71, 72, 73, 74, 77, 93, 96,
97, 98, 99, 102, 107, 108, 115,
117, 119, 121, 125, 135, 138,
139, 143, 148, 153, 154, 156,
158, 163, 165, 166, 167, 168,
169, 173, 177, 178, 179, 180,
188, 202, 203, 204, 209
Mitrovich, Luke, 143, 203
Mitrovich, Marissa, 15, 25, 26, 32,
108, 158, 166, 179, 180
Mitrovich, Tim, 158
Monetti, Thomas W., 121, 136
Morley Field, 36
Morrison, Mary 157, 158
Morse, Guy, 200
Mtolo, Willie, 124
Muhrcke, Gary, 124
Munk, Gary, 128
Muno, Rich, 206
Murphy, Tim, 121
Mwakawago, Daudi N., 121

N

Neiman, Janet, 142
Neiman, LeRoy, 121, 142, 178, 184,
208
Newark International Airport, 110, 116
New York City Marathon
1970, 33
1978, 85
1980, 86
1985, 12

219

"After spending eighteen years in the US Senate trying to solve many problems for this fine country of ours, I thought I knew "the ropes"—but after watching my friend Dan Mitrovich try to get a statue in New York's Central Park, my efforts were "kid stuff!" After reading this wonderful book about Dan's courage and persistence, you'll know one thing for sure: there is a statue of Fred Lebow in Central Park! Here you will read what it takes to overcome huge obstacles in a quest to accomplish something of great good."

—Alan K. Simpson, United States Senator, Wyoming (retired)

"It is an inspiring story of a man whose remarkable level of determination and ingenuity enabled him to complete a most ambitious undertaking... If you want to be encouraged about your fellow man, this is a good book to read."

—Ronald F. Phillips, Senior Vice Chancellor & School of Law Dean Emeritus, Pepperdine University

"A perfect ending to a life well run, and a must-read for any fan of our sport—not just running, but any sport."

—Tracy Sundlun, Senior VP of Global Events for the Competitor Group and Co-Founder of the Rock'n'Roll Marathon Series

"Fred Lebow was an amazing man, the founding father of the New York City Marathon. It took another amazing man, Dan Mitrovich, to have Fred's statue created and then placed in Central Park. This is the compelling story of these two visionaries."

—George A. Hirsch, chairman of the New York Road Runners Club and former worldwide publisher of *Runner's World*